'There is an increasing number of adults who have a diagnosis of Asperger syndrome in their mature years. This new book will help explain past experiences, provide self-understanding and give guidance as to the future. People who have recently achieved a diagnosis, family members and clinicians will find the descriptions and advice invaluable.'

– Tony Attwood, PhD, Clinical Psychologist, Minds & Hearts Clinic, Australia, and author of The Complete Guide to Asperger's Syndrome

'Philip Wylie has captured the true essence of living with Asperger syndrome. Many people spend the majority of their lives wondering why they are different and never fit in. Broken relationships, loss of jobs, and being preyed upon by those who see our vulnerability and lack of assertiveness are all part of the process. In turn, we develop low self-esteem and suffer many consequences. Getting diagnosed can help turn these negatives into positives. No matter how late in life you discover that you have Asperger's, there is still room for repair. Wylie points out that receiving a diagnosis can have either positive or negative effects, and what to be prepared for in either case. Self-acceptance is the key. You are then free to embark upon a new life. Within these pages is advice for what happens next after receiving your diagnosis. Wylie helps guide you through the process, to come out seeing the light at the end of the tunnel. That light will help guide you to a better life after learning you are on the autism spectrum!'

– Anita Lesko, Founder and Executive Director of the Flying High with Autism Foundation, editor of Been There. Done That. Try This! *and author of* Asperger's Syndrome: When Life Hands You Lemons, Make Lemonade

'A timely accurate resource for discovering if you fit the bill for autism. How I wish this treasure of a resource had been available during my own journey! This important guide for adults cuts to the chase. It potentially opens all the right doors.'

— *Wenn Lawson, Psychologist, Counsellor, Social Worker, author and autism advocate*

VERY LATE DIAGNOSIS OF ASPERGER SYNDROME (AUTISM SPECTRUM DISORDER)

of related interest

The Complete Guide to Asperger's Syndrome
Tony Attwood
ISBN 978 1 84310 495 7 (hardback)
ISBN 978 1 84310 669 2 (paperback)
eISBN 978 1 84642 559 2

Coming Out Asperger
Diagnosis, Disclosure and Self-Confidence
Edited by Dinah Murray
ISBN 978 1 84310 240 3
eISBN 978 1 84642 450 2

Been There. Done That. Try This!
An Aspie's Guide to Life on Earth
Edited by Tony Attwood, Craig R. Evans and Anita Lesko
ISBN 978 1 84905 964 0
eISBN 978 0 85700 871 8

Asperger Syndrome and Anxiety
A Guide to Successful Stress Management
Nick Dubin
Foreword by Valerie Gaus
ISBN 978 1 84310 895 5
eISBN 978 1 84642 922 4

The Autism Spectrum and Depression
Nick Dubin
Foreword by Tony Attwood
ISBN 978 1 84905 814 8
eISBN 978 0 85700 242 6

AutiPower!
Successful Living and Working with an Autism Spectrum Disorder
Herman Jansen and Betty Rombout
ISBN 978 1 84905 437 9
eISBN 978 0 85700 869 5

VERY LATE DIAGNOSIS OF ASPERGER SYNDROME (AUTISM SPECTRUM DISORDER)

How Seeking a Diagnosis in Adulthood Can Change Your Life

PHILIP WYLIE
Forewords by Luke Beardon and Sara Heath

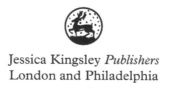

Jessica Kingsley *Publishers*
London and Philadelphia

The Autism Spectrum Quotient (AQ) in the Appendix is reproduced from Baron-Cohen *et al.* 2001 with the kind permission of the Autism Research Centre at Cambridge.

First published in 2014
by Jessica Kingsley Publishers
73 Collier Street
London N1 9BE, UK
and
400 Market Street, Suite 400
Philadelphia, PA 19106, USA

www.jkp.com

Library of Congress Cataloging in Publication Data
A CIP catalog record for this book is available from the Library of Congress

British Library Cataloguing in Publication Data
A CIP catalogue record for this book is available from the British Library

ISBN 978 1 84905 433 1
eISBN 978 0 85700 778 0

Printed and bound in Great Britain

To the well-being and independence
of late-diagnosed autistic adults

DISCLAIMER

Asperger syndrome, which has been reclassified as autism spectrum disorder (ASD) by the American Psychiatric Association in the fifth edition of the *Diagnostic and Statistical Manual of Mental Disorders (DSM-5)*, is a highly diverse neurological condition that affects individuals in many different ways. The characteristics of ASD – both gifts and impairments – vary massively, so not all of the information in this guide will be applicable to everyone. This book applies to the late diagnosis of potentially hidden neurological conditions, including Asperger syndrome (ASD). The diagnosis, which follows self-identification, is potentially lethal without accompanying psychological, emotional and financial support; however, with adequate and appropriate support, a diagnosis can positively change your life.

CONTENTS

FOREWORD

Getting a diagnosis of Asperger syndrome (AS) or autism can be a traumatic time for many people – it can also be a joyful time, a time of relief, of sudden epiphany-esque understanding, the starting point of a bereavement process, or absolute mystification. It can even be a combination of all of these. However, what has been rarely investigated is what a diagnosis (or, as I prefer it, identification) of AS means to someone who has already lived most of their life, and has 'stumbled' across their identity very late on in life.

An identification of AS can mean so many different things to so many people; indeed, it would seem sensible to suggest that the heterogeneity of the population is such that each person will react in his or her own, unique, manner. However, this does not detract from what Philip has set out to do in this book, which is to identify many of the common themes that are associated with a very late diagnosis of Asperger syndrome. While not all of these themes and not all of the content will be 100 per cent pertinent to every reader, there is an excellent chance that much of what has been written will be applicable to most – especially those who themselves have had a very late diagnosis of AS.

Asperger syndrome is extraordinarily misunderstood. It is often very misunderstood by clinical professionals, and is often very misunderstood by the general public. This can cause immense distress to so many individuals who have AS, not least in their struggle to get a formal identification. Not all people who get a very late diagnosis will have gone through a struggle to actually get a confirmed diagnosis, but I suspect a lot will. This, in itself, is harmful for many people – along with many of the diagnostic practices that can be patronizing, demeaning, medically based, and all about identifying weaknesses or 'impairments'. The post-diagnostic support should be part of the diagnostic process itself. Anyone involved in the diagnostic pathway should be treating the individual with the respect they deserve, as opposed to as a 'patient' who needs 'assessing'. Ascertaining whether an individual has the fascinating cognitive style associated with AS should be a privilege – and diagnosticians should take note of that fact. Sadly, this is not often the case, and individuals are made to feel somehow less of a human being. This has huge implications for how a diagnosis is subsequently dealt with by the individual. Indeed, for someone who has spent most of his or her life without a diagnosis, it could be argued that this identification process should be handled with even greater sensitivity than with anyone else. Again, sadly, this is not always the case.

Many individuals who end up with a very late diagnosis of AS will have had problems with their mental health. This is indicative of how poor societies in general are at understanding, supporting and making adjustments for differing cognitive styles, which then leads on to feelings of poor self-esteem, and, sometimes, major problems such as depression for the individual. How mental health is then reacted to by the professionals involved is of paramount importance. To 'treat' mental ill health without relating it to the AS is a dangerous game to play. AS will have a huge impact on the individual, and must be taken into account. I believe that with the appropriate post-diagnostic support many individuals with AS will have such a better understanding of self that issues with mental health can decrease dramatically. It is essential, therefore, that after identification the individual has the support required to assist him or her to have a better understanding of self and, subsequently, improved self-esteem. So many individuals will have gone through life blaming themselves for all sorts of problems; this is such a common theme among the unidentified population, as well as those who have had a late diagnosis. It is imperative that those individuals are allowed to understand why life has been the way that it has for them, and that many of the problems that they have had actually relate to other people's poor understanding of them, as opposed to the blame being theirs.

There are bound to be aspects of Philip's book that do not apply to all individuals with AS, diagnosed or not, late diagnosed or not. However, what he has done is create a set of components that are very well worth considering in relation to a late diagnosis. Having AS can be a complicated enough part of life to learn how to deal with at any age. To be identified late in life is bound to add complications that an earlier identification might have avoided. As the world is very gradually getting better (though is a very long way off from optimal practice) at identifying individuals with autism/AS, it is to be expected that more adults will be gaining a very late diagnosis. I am aware of some excellent clinical practice in the diagnosis of autism/AS, but suspect that there is still some way to go. My opinions are based on numerous self-reported examples from within the UK.

It is essential that the issues surrounding a very late diagnosis are explored thoroughly, and support made available to ensure that individuals are not let down. Philip has made an excellent start in identifying many of those issues.

Dr Luke Beardon

FOREWORD

This book is important. There is much written about Asperger syndrome (ASD) but little from the perspective of very late diagnosis and the problems this causes people of middle and later ages who have known that they are different, but not the reasons why this is so.

I am very pleased to have met Phil, as it was our initial contact via email that set the seeds for our interesting research project, the *VLDAS 2013 UK Survey*, which I hope will be one of many. The project evolved from a short, cryptic email from Phil in 2012 in which he was seeking non-clinical acknowledgement and recognition that he had Asperger syndrome (ASD) and requesting my help and support. I guided and mentored him on his self-realisation journey, and his ASD 'coming in' and 'coming out', which surprisingly led to the birth of this book.

Thanks to Phil's book, we have a much better chance to raise the profile of autism in older people (and there are still many who sadly remain undiagnosed), and to recognise it in them and talk about it. Phil's story and his useful self-help strategies will now help other mature adults gain insight into themselves as well as understand and cope better with their issues.

My personal view is that Asperger syndrome (ASD) is not a disability but different wiring in the brain and a wish to live a more ordered life. Asperger syndrome (ASD) is not a mental health condition but a different culture, and part of the diversity of humanity. I embrace the skills and talents of the many mature adults who, with the help of this book, will now embark and progress on their diagnostic journey, as they have skills, imagination and expertise about which I can only dream.

Sara Heath MEd
Founder and Director, Shropshire Autonomy

ACKNOWLEDGEMENTS

Special thanks to the following professional autism specialists, psychologists and other relevant practitioners who have kindly contributed to this guidebook:

Maxine Aston is a BACP-accredited counsellor and has an MSc in Health Psychology. She is qualified as a supervisor and trainer, and as a teacher in adult education. Maxine runs her own counselling centre where her specialisation is working with individuals, couples and families affected by Asperger syndrome (ASD). Maxine is the author of four books about relationships and dating for adults who are on the spectrum. She also provides ASD assessments and relationship workshops. Further information is available at www.maxineaston.co.uk.

Tony Attwood PhD is a clinical psychologist who has specialised in autism spectrum disorders, and especially Asperger syndrome, for over 30 years. He is an adjunct professor at Griffith University and is the chairperson at the Minds and Hearts Clinic in Brisbane (www. mindsandhearts.net). He works as a clinician and is the author of several books on Asperger syndrome, including *Asperger's Syndrome: A Guide for Parents and Professionals*, which has sold over 400,000 copies, and *The Complete Guide to Asperger's Syndrome*. Further information is available at www.tonyattwood.com.au.

Luke Beardon BA (Hons), PG Cert (Autism), EdD is a senior lecturer in autism at Sheffield Hallam University. He has worked with the National Autistic Society as a trainer and consultant, as well as a service coordinator in residential services, helping young autistic adults to access suitable residential services. Luke works in various capacities, from consultant to researcher and trainer. He has also written, edited and provided forewords for several publications about autism and Asperger syndrome. He is also a registered expert witness (see www.the-expert-witness.co.uk/luke-beardon). His doctor of education thesis is on 'Asperger Syndrome and Perceived Offending Conduct'.

Jen Birch is a New Zealander who was diagnosed with Asperger syndrome at the age of 43. Jen wrote her book, *Congratulations! It's Asperger Syndrome* in 2003 and participated in a documentary about Asperger syndrome entitled, 'Life Among Strangers'. More information can be found on her website (www.aspergers.co.nz).

Michael John Carley became aware of his Aspergic condition at the age of 36, shortly after his son's diagnosis. Later, in 2003, Michael founded the New York-based not-for-profit Global and Regional Asperger Syndrome Partnership (GRASP). Since its inception, GRASP's chapter organisation has grown to provide 27 facilitated support groups for people on the autism spectrum across the United States and Canada. Michael is executive director of GRASP and its sister organisation, the Asperger Syndrome Training and Employment Partnership (ASTEP), which provides training and consultancy for employers and educates them about the benefits and limitations of employing people on the autism spectrum.

Michael Fitzgerald MD, MB, Bch, BAO, DObst, DPM, FRC, Psych, MRCS (Eng), MInst Psychoanal is Henry Marsh Professor of Child and Adolescent Psychiatry at Trinity College Dublin. He was the first Professor of Child Psychiatry in Ireland in 1996. He has a doctorate in autism. He trained at St Patrick's Hospital Dublin, Chicago Medical School and the Maudsley Hospital. He has clinically diagnosed over 2600 individuals with autism and Asperger syndrome and has served on the Government Task Force on Autism and the Family. His website address is www.professormichaelfitzgerald.eu.

Sara Heath MEd is a believer in the social model of disability. She established Autonomy (see www.shropshireautonomy.co.uk), an Asperger syndrome self-help group based in Shropshire, and runs it with her son, Eric. Sara is also a practitioner at AutonomyPlus+, an Asperger-specific consultancy, where she provides pre-diagnostic assessments and reports for people on the autism spectrum, as well as post-diagnostic support services. Sara interviewed the survey respondents, who are all national or local members of Autonomy, for the *VLDAS 2013 UK Survey*, which she published jointly with Philip Wylie. Sara has a Cert Ed in Special Needs from Westhill College, Birmingham, an MEd in Exceptional Children from the University of Georgia, Athens, GA, an Advanced Certificate in Dyslexia accredited by the BDA, and a postgraduate certificate in Business (Social Enterprise).

Sarah Hendrickx is an independent specialist consultant, trainer and coach in autism spectrum conditions. Sarah delivers training across the UK to improve understanding and support for those with autism spectrum conditions. Diagnosed with Asperger syndrome (ASD) at the age of 41, it took Sarah many years of working within the field of autism – including having five books published and completing an MA in Autism – before realising that the reason that she understood it so well was that she had it herself. Sarah speaks at conferences about her own experience of autism. Her website address is www.asperger-training.com.

Debra Moore PhD is a psychologist and director of Fall Creek Counseling Associates, a private practice serving Sacramento and Placer counties in California, USA (see www.sacramentopsychology.com). She has been in practice since the early 1980s and has enjoyed seeing clients, managing Fall Creek, and mentoring and supervising psychology students and therapists in training. Debra's goal is to provide quality, accessible psychotherapy and consultation, to educate the public about psychology and mental health through her website and public speaking, and to provide quality training to interns.

Rod Morris is co-founder of the UK autistic-led not-for-profit social enterprise WASP with Asperger Limited (see www.wasp.uk.com). He is also co-author of the book, *Asperger's for Professionals*. His diagnosed neurological profile includes autism, dyslexia, dyscalculia and dyspraxia with a 'unique and complex form of intelligence'. Having gained a BA in Media, a PGCE, and a postgraduate certificate in Asperger syndrome, he is currently studying for an MA in Autism at Sheffield Hallam University, with a view to following up with a PhD. His most recent work includes delivery of workshops to one of the largest local authorities in Europe, a proposal for the development of a Royal College of Autism and the design of a unique service model.

Altazar Rossiter PhD is a shamanic 'healer' who provides coaching programmes, workshops and consultations for developing spiritual and emotional intelligence (see www.altazarrossiter.com). Altazar's doctorate is in Semiotics, which covers symbolism and psychoanalytic theory. His book is entitled *Developing Spiritual Intelligence: The Power of You*, published by O Books in 2006. Altazar believes that we are all here for a purpose, so he is passionate about enabling his clients to find their own way – whether that fits the norm of the social order or not – and to be at peace with themselves in their unique way.

Thanks also to the following Aspergic people who kindly agreed to be included in the book as case studies:

Wendy Lim and **8Ball** are profiled fully in Luke Beardon's book, *Aspies on Mental Health*, published by Jessica Kingsley Publishers.

Sarah McCulloch was diagnosed in the UK at the age of 23. She works with digital media and is also a freelance writer and copy editor (see www.sarahmcculloch.com).

Roderick Wintour was born in 1962 in West Auckland, New Zealand and diagnosed at the age of 31. In 1998, he founded the New Zealand Aspire trust to support students with ASD and associated disorders in education. He introduced ASD awareness to many different schools in New Zealand and was the first ASD public speaker in his country. For 11 years, he worked on health and education teams in many schools and working with the most challenging cases. Roderick has also been a strong supporter and volunteer of ASD research and is well known for his ASD poetry and articles.

Other contributors

I thank the members of Autonomy Shropshire (including Carol-Anne, John Carlisle, Fred Smith and Chris Stevens) who voluntarily participated in the *VLDAS 2013 UK Survey* (Wylie and Heath 2013). (Please refer to the Introduction for information about this survey.) I also thank Simon Baron-Cohen and the researchers at the Autism Research Centre at the University of Cambridge for giving us their kind permission to reproduce the Autism Quotient (AQ) test in the Appendix, as well as Emily McClave and her colleagues at Jessica Kingsley Publishers for their guidance and will to make this book successful.

PREFACE

I would like to share with you the experiences which led to my formal diagnosis of Asperger syndrome (ASD) in 2013.

I always knew that I was different but did not understand the underlying cause. I always struggled to maintain relationships and jobs, and for decades I was unaware of the severe stress and social anxiety I was experiencing. Shortly after I completed my first degree, I consulted a firm of educational psychologists who identified my high level of anxiety. Naturally, I was worried, but unfortunately I was unable to discuss these matters in my family and I distrusted psychiatric medicine; therefore, I adopted the 'do-it-yourself' approach: I subscribed to *Psychology Today* magazine and learned about natural medicine. I tried hard to fit in, but if my ability to fit in was to be measured by my income, my attempts to mimic neurotypical people were unsuccessful. I did, however, qualify as a chartered accountant after studying for an MBA in London, and I systemised many businesses as either finance manager, systems accountant or finance director. Unfortunately, I could not manage my stress levels or earn enough income, so in 2003 I left the UK to live in northern Thailand.

During the subsequent ten years in Southeast Asia I was on a quest to understand myself. Indirectly, I identified my neurological condition by systemising my life. The result of my self-systemisation is a developmental model for late diagnosis of ASD known as the Nine Degrees of Autism. Tony Attwood commented on this model, 'I think it is intuitively appealing but also clinically fairly accurate from people I have known' (Attwood 2013). I am currently seeking funding for a doctorate to enable scientific validation of this developmental model.

In November 2011, at the age of 51, I discovered my latent 'intellectual condition' in Phnom Penh, Cambodia. One morning, I was browsing through my professional *Accountancy* magazine and read an excellent article about autism by Mark Lever, CEO of the National Autistic Society (Lever 2011). Alarm bells rang and I knew I would have to face a very inconvenient truth. Although I received a positive pre-diagnostic ASD assessment in 2012, I had to wait until 2013 before I received a formal diagnosis by a registered psychiatrist.

Once I became aware of my condition, I researched everything related to Asperger syndrome (ASD). Although I experienced a painful and traumatic crisis, I knew that I had reached an important milestone in my journey of self-enquiry. At last, my life began to make sense! Now I understood why I had always had relationship problems both inside and outside my family. It explained to some extent why I was constructively dismissed by the firm of accountants for which I had worked. It also made sense of the fact that so many people had described me as being strange, eccentric, interesting, ungrounded, uncoordinated, selfish and so forth.

For many years, I had been aware that I was a thinker, an intellectual and, above all, an individual. I had to do things my way and I always questioned illogical rules. I upset many authority figures over the years, beginning with my father.

My adept ability to memorise information was my undoing. I passed examinations with ease and believed that I was more intelligent than many other people. I wrongly attributed my 'differences' to superior intelligence and an enlightened mindset. When I realised that I was autistic, my castle sank into the quicksand. I soon grasped, however, that my traits and eccentric ways were shared by over 1 per cent of the population. Now I understood why I could not survive in an office environment for long, and why so many people misunderstood me. But, on the bright side, I had found the key to my life.

Now I am much clearer about my strengths and weaknesses than before my diagnosis. My experience of self-identification has not been easy, however. As my mentor, Sara Heath, commented:

I think you now know – and wish you did not know – that you have ASD. Some people are set free by a diagnosis to be who they really are, but others need some downtime to process the change and come to terms with it, as you do. Let time do its work.

I experienced a mental breakdown when I discovered my autistic condition. I had run out of money and was experiencing horrendous employment issues. I could not see a way forward. For the first time in my life, I felt truly desperate and suicidal. Now I am a different and much more grounded person, and even my values and interests have changed.

Before self-identification of my condition, my journey of self-enquiry had been very thorough indeed:

- I consulted psychics, healers, spiritual gurus in India, numerologists, psychotherapists, psychologists, fortune tellers, shamans, hypnotists, personal development cults, bodywork practitioners and faith healers in the Philippines.

- I trained as a civil engineer, salesman, chartered accountant, auditor, tax advisor, aromatherapist, numerologist, Neuro-Linguistic Programming (NLP) practitioner, workshop facilitator, lecturer, Reiki healer and Lightbody Integration practitioner, among other 'careers'.

- I worked for hundreds of organisations in numerous positions, including builder's gofer, barman, company director, company secretary and head of group administration of a private British bank.

- I studied the metaphysics of transformation with numerology and geometry. I also studied Jungian psychology, alchemy and other metaphysical systems such as the Enneagram and the Kabbalah.

Perhaps it's ironic that my soul-searching was so extensive, as I found my answer accidentally in a magazine article. I am grateful to my godfather for showing me the path of ASD in my family.

An important aspect of my healing process was understanding the family genetics behind it.

I hope that you enjoy, learn and grow by reading this book. Please understand that I wrote this book during my identity-alignment breakdown, from which I have since recovered. Now I would like to help fellow adults who have ASD to have a great life!

Philip Wylie
www.phil.asia
www.ninedegrees.pw

INTRODUCTION

This book is about the personal transformation that follows very late diagnosis of autism spectrum disorder (VLDASD) – previously classified as Asperger syndrome – and is for adults who are on the autism spectrum (pre- and post-diagnosis), their families, professional carers and students of this, as yet, not fully understood intellectual condition.

The autistic adult's personal transformation typically begins with feeling different during childhood and continues beyond the dates of self-identification and diagnosis of ASD until the individual fully accepts his or her new identity. This book not only looks at these issues, but goes further by providing practical guidance about living authentically and harmoniously as an autistic individual after accepting our new 'self'.

The uniqueness of this book

There are good essays available on various aspects of the process of coming to terms with the diagnosis of ASD, but this is the first book that clearly and chronologically outlines the whole tumultuous path. If soon-to-be or recently diagnosed individuals have at least some idea of what lies ahead of them, sharing with the many others who have also gone through this, the process will be eased. (Carley 2008, Introduction)

Hence, this book is different by design. There are many interesting autobiographies out there, written mainly by recently diagnosed autistic adults who had adequate love and support in their lives. This book is for a wider audience because I and others in some of the case studies included herein experienced a turbulent post-diagnostic journey with minimal support.

This book is a guidebook rather than an autobiography, and is intended for an international audience because I received valuable contributions from all over the world. It also contains enlightening insights from a UK survey of 20 late-diagnosed autistic adults that I conducted and published with Sara Heath from AutonomyPlus+ (Wylie and Heath 2013). Our survey, which covers many aspects of the post-diagnostic identity alignment process, is a great source of information both quantitatively in the statistics it provides and qualitatively in the personal experiences it records. Every autistic adult's diagnostic experience is unique, so it is important to draw upon as many case studies as possible.

Throughout my post-self-identification identity crisis I consulted my mentor, Sara Heath, as well as other autism specialists, psychologists, psychiatrists, carers and healers. So this guidebook is the result of my collaboration with some of the world's top autism researchers and other relevant experts. The inclusion of scientific findings means that this book achieves a harmonious balance between theory and practice.

I supplemented scientific research with alternative ideas and practices. I am not limited by any academic regime, research institution or orthodox system (although I do have a Master's degree in management science), so I am free to dig in uncharted territory without any limitations. Like many people who have ASD, I value freedom, autonomy and independent thinking, and I am inclined towards natural medicine (rather than psychiatry) whenever feasible.

Unfortunately, there is an abundance of misinformation – peppered with disinformation – on the subject of ASD. It would not be fair to expect the public to understand the nature of autism while the medical profession is itself still struggling to understand this often hidden intellectual disability. This book, therefore, questions the efficacy of some of the existing diagnostic systems and treatments, and highlights several myths related to the autism spectrum.

This is a work of 'involuntary investigative journalism' undertaken while I was compelled to understand my intellectual condition. Not to put too fine a point on it, this project may have saved my life, and I hope that this guidebook will help many other adults as they discover the underlying cause of some of the ASD difficulties that they have experienced in their life.

The psychiatrists' 'bible', the *Diagnostic and Statistical Manual of Mental Disorders*, published by the American Psychiatric Association (APA) and now in its fifth edition (*DSM-5*; APA 2013), lists hundreds of mental disorders and their diagnostic criteria; however, the publication lists negative criteria only.

An alternative viewpoint is that high-functioning autism includes a triad of the following gifts:

- ability to focus on a task for a long period of time

- above-average intelligence with adept logical reasoning ability

- ability to understand and simplify complex sets of data.

An estimated 1 per cent of the global population is on the autism spectrum, and the prevalence of autism is growing. It is helpful to understand the history of scientific research into Asperger syndrome as it explains why so many Aspergic adults remain undiagnosed. Although Leo Kanner and Hans Asperger published research papers about classic autism and 'autistic psychopathy' in 1943 and 1944, respectively, Asperger's work was referred to but not actually translated into the English language until 1989 (Frith 1991); therefore, the majority of English-speaking doctors and autism practitioners would not have been aware of what was originally known as 'Asperger's disorder' until the 1990s. Then, when funding became available for screening and diagnosis of autism, the money was allocated primarily for children, so autistic adults were left at the back of the queue.

Screening of children for ASD began in many developed countries in the 1990s, so any adults at that time missed the opportunity of diagnostic support; therefore, many undiagnosed or late-diagnosed autistic individuals are over 40 years old. For diagnosis to be effective, appropriate and timely intervention is necessary; otherwise, mental health issues are likely to emerge. Late diagnosis often occurs whenever additional health issues are caused by the delay of suitable intervention. If we adopt this latter definition of 'late diagnosis', even young children can be included.

What is late diagnosis of Asperger syndrome?

Tony Attwood offers the following perspective on late diagnosis of Asperger syndrome:

> I think that the person themselves will have noticed that they were different many years ago and the adjustment strategies could either have been constructive or destructive psychologically. Very late diagnosis of Asperger syndrome (ASD), from my perspective, really refers to those who may be middle-aged or older who, to a certain extent, have adjusted to or camouflaged the characteristics of Asperger syndrome (ASD). I do recognise that some with Asperger syndrome (ASD) can socialise very well, but it's at the cost of intellectual and emotional exhaustion, and this can confuse others in terms of sometimes seeing social competence but other times seeing a great need for social withdrawal and isolation. The advantage of a late diagnostic assessment can be that it will explain many aspects of the person's developmental history from bullying and teasing to issues in relation to emotion management and relationships. In general, those who have been diagnosed later in life have been very pleased to have that diagnosis as a means of explaining being different. It can also be useful in terms of the future in focusing on strengths rather than trying to resolve weaknesses. (Tony Attwood, personal correspondence, 16 October 2013)

Michael Fitzgerald offers this comment:

> ASD should be screened in children by the age of 12–13 years (at the latest, during the first year at secondary school). I diagnose ASD from the age of 4 years upwards. I diagnose adults up into their sixties, and most have been misdiagnosed as having schizophrenia. (Michael Fitzgerald, interview, 10 October 2013)

In the 1960s and 1970s, treatments for autism were experimental by nature, ranging from psychedelic drugs (including LSD) to electric shock treatment and behavioural therapy. Behavioural therapy is based on the premise that autism can be 'cured' by encouraging patients to act 'normally'. 'Good behaviour' is rewarded, while 'bad behaviour' results in punishment – just like in Pavlov's experiments with dogs. Unfortunately, this 'medical model' often causes autistic individuals to have low self-esteem and mental ill health.

In view of the treatments available to autistic people during the 1960s and 1970s, due to a misunderstanding of the condition, it is not surprising that many autistic adults and their families avoided psychiatric treatment at all costs. This may well be one of the reasons for the high prevalence of undiagnosed autistic adults.

Neurologically, there are many reasons why late-diagnosed autistic adults are more complex than children, and the post-diagnostic identity crisis is potentially much more severe. Also, autistic adults, who often have no family or carer, are the last people to receive any support; therefore, to answer this need, I have covered the main pitfalls that autistic adults can encounter, and offered as much practical advice as possible.

I sincerely hope that the guidance in this book will improve the lives of autistic adults and break down existing barriers between the neurotypical majority and the emerging autistic population around the world. Although our strengths are many and we have a lot to offer society, the world at large has a long way to go in understanding and accepting neurodiversity. Here are a number of questions to contemplate:

- Since we know that autism is primarily inherited genetically, why do people fund research into the 'cause' of autism?

- Why is there talk about 'cures' for ASD when we cannot change this condition that we were born with, and many autistic adults wouldn't want to be 'normal' ('neurotypical') anyway?

- Why are official diagnoses for ASD often provided by practitioners who have minimal specialist training in this disability, thereby causing a frighteningly high rate of misdiagnosis?

- Given that autistic individuals have achieved some of the greatest feats in history, why are we not valued more by society?

- If autism social enterprises and charities are intended to benefit autistic people, why don't they employ more people who are on the autism spectrum?

- If society were more tolerant of 'neurodiversity', wouldn't a greater proportion of the growing ASD community be more productive and therefore beneficial to the economy?

- Wouldn't it be more beneficial for society to accept neurological differences instead of coercing people into expressing themselves inauthentically?

Chapter 1

THE STAGES OF VERY LATE DIAGNOSIS OF AUTISM SPECTRUM DISORDER

This chapter outlines the key stages before, during and after the very late diagnosis of autism spectrum disorder (VLDASD) that will be addressed in subsequent chapters. These stages are:

- knowing that we are different

- getting external feedback and clues that we have ASD

- pretending to be normal (and possibly resisting self-identification due to fear of the mental health system and the stigma of disability)

- reaching the 'tipping point' of self-identification (acknowledgement of ASD), which may involve experiencing 'meltdowns', trauma and crisis, or relief

- researching ASD and reaching self-discovery (with authoritative sources of information)

- receiving a pre-diagnostic assessment and a diagnosis of ASD

- 'coming out' and deciding in whom to confide

- finding self-acceptance through enhanced understanding of our strengths (or gifts)

- enjoying a sustainable future (with adequate income, special interests and satisfying relationships).

Although the above stages are listed in a logical order, in practice the sequence of events may differ, and some processes may occur simultaneously. There is not a 'one size fits all' diagnostic template for all those who find themselves on the autism spectrum; each person's diagnostic journey is unique. Autistic people are not always teased at school, or bullied at work, and some have supportive families. Also, people react in many different ways to their diagnosis, so this chapter simply describes a 'typical VLDASD journey' while providing useful guidance and cautionary notes.

Knowing that we are different

Most autistic adults who are diagnosed late in their lives say that they always knew they were different, but they did not understand how or why until the 'tipping point' of self-identification.

> This usually occurs between the ages of six and eight years old. Until then, the differences are gender and race. Now the difference is ability and personality. (Tony Attwood, interview, 13 November 2013)

The following quote is typical of our survey respondents: 'I knew I was different but I did not know why, so I felt relief (after the diagnosis) because I wanted to know the reason why' (Wylie and Heath 2013, p.22). During the early stage of development, the autistic child may or may not look normal or tend to appear or act like 'Joe 90' or a 'little professor' who constantly asks questions, which may seem both naïve and annoying, especially to his or her parents. This child's mind is highly logical, so the use of 'systemisation' (a form of mental curiosity that seeks to understand the relationships between 'things') is common. On the other hand, this child's emotions may be 'numb' and confusing.

> Knowing that I was different to other people, but not knowing why, has done serious damage, and possibly irreparable damage to my self-esteem… Nobody, whether disabled or otherwise, comes into the world with poor self-esteem. The damage is

done by other people through their attitudes and their reactions to us. (Beardon 2011, p.142)

Most people on the autism spectrum who are diagnosed late in life had a bewildering childhood without understanding why they appeared weird to other people, or why they were treated differently from 'normal' people. Some autistic children are teased and bullied at school and/or psychologically abused or neglected at home. The lucky ones have parents who genuinely love and care for them, and provide the special education and support (assuming they have the means) that they need to succeed.

Many of the problems that autistic people have stem from our logical minds that have difficulty understanding and accepting illogical social norms, written and unwritten rules, and fashion statements. Our direct and honest comments may seem abrasive, but we do not intend to cause an argument or hurt another person's feelings. As a result of each misunderstanding or argument, our self-esteem takes a knock, so, if we are diagnosed very late in life, it is likely that in the meantime we will have experienced mental ill health and developed low self-esteem; therefore, obtaining a diagnosis as early as possible would normally benefit our well-being.

Getting external feedback and clues that we have ASD

Unfortunately, most of the external feedback offered to autistic people is negative and includes teasing, ridicule, bullying, exclusion from social groups and so forth. A characteristic of animals, including human beings, is fear of the unknown, and usually fear provokes aggressive behaviour and victimisation of 'the threat'. So the boy who is scared of wasps wants to kill them, while children who notice an alien-like being in their presence tend to instigate 'us versus them' enemy patterning.

Autistic people think and behave differently compared with neurotypical people. These differences may seem eccentric or very strange. For example, the autistic person may have a strange cackle of a laugh that draws the attention of bystanders, or they may have trouble with what most people consider simple tasks. People who have ASD can often solve the most complex problems but struggle with some relatively simple tasks. We may also have impaired motor skills and issues with coordination, making us easy targets for bullies.

Those of us who are diagnosed as having ASD late in life have probably received hundreds of clues related to our condition without understanding their significance. The significance of the following list of clues, descriptions which may apply to you, may be meaningful after several decades of confusion and humiliation. Please be aware that each of the descriptive 'clues' below are negative, and therefore identification with these labels over several decades will have inevitably damaged our self-esteem.

- *Selfish:* Autistic people are self-absorbed in intellectual 'bubbles' and may spurn social events or group activities which make us feel uncomfortable. Autism derives from the Greek word *autos*, which means 'self'. We are driven by our special interests, so our behaviour may seem selfish or aloof.

- *Clumsy:* Many autistic people are less coordinated than neurotypical people, so there are not many top sportspeople in the autism community, particularly in the realm of team sports. This is unfortunate because many people consider participation in team sports and keeping abreast of national soccer or rugby leagues as mandatory for 'normal' men.

- *Mad:* Sometimes the combination of creativity, eccentricity, anger and mental ill health is incorrectly perceived as madness, or labelled as schizophrenia; however, most of us are simply quirky because we lack the ongoing reality checks to which neurotypical people have access.

- *Alien:* Sometimes people who are on the autism spectrum are regarded as aliens from another planet because our ways are different, and sometimes taboo or even offensive. Jen Birch says in her book that one of her identity issues was, 'Am I an earthling or an alien?' (Birch 2003, p.46).

- *Naïve:* Many people who have ASD are easily tricked and manipulated due to our lack of cognitive empathy (our ability to perceive other people's thoughts and feelings). Another term for cognitive empathy is 'theory of mind'.

- *Ungrounded:* Many autistic people tend to be intellectual thinkers lacking man-management and executive skills as well as basic coping skills that facilitate survival; however, the good news is that diagnosis helps us to ground ourselves and become more practical.

Pretending to be normal and possibly resisting self-identification

One way to survive in a predominantly neurotypical world is to act like a neurotypical (normal) person, and many autistic adults do so for decades before we finally understand ourselves; however, pretending to be someone else damages our self-esteem and mental health because we feel unable to honour and express ourselves truthfully.

Pretending to be normal is a common survival strategy for many people on the autism spectrum. We know that we are more likely to get a job if we improve our presentation or when we boast about our achievements. We want our interviewer or potential boss to tick all of the recruitment check boxes, but we also want him or her to like us, so by using 'small talk' and a little humour, we improve our chances of success.

> Children try to fit in after the age of eight. Before that, they may have been isolated, but now the person tries to fit in and uses different ways from observation, imitation and so forth. The self-identification and diagnosis can be when the person has the mental maturity to understand the actual terms and diagnosis. But what I tend to find is that teenagers don't want the diagnosis – not because they disagree with diagnosis itself but rather fear that diagnosis will lead to victimisation. They know that their peers view anyone who has a disorder in a derogatory way. (Tony Attwood, interview, 13 November 2013)

Another negative consequence of pretending to be normal is increased stress, anxiety and mental exhaustion. Acting in real life is a stressful occupation, and although there may be material benefits, there are plenty of negative mental and emotional repercussions.

While we pretend to be normal we are denying our condition. In our survey, 25 per cent of the respondents admitted that they had denied their condition (Wylie and Heath 2013).

Fred Smith states:

> For a long time I felt things would be better if I could 'just pull myself together' but unfortunately this increased my feelings of depression and anxiety because I was putting on a front and trying to mask my symptoms. (Wylie and Heath 2013, p.20)

Some of us try to hide our condition because we are scared of psychiatry, mental health treatments and psychiatric hospitals. Our survey provides evidence that many autistic adults distrust psychiatry and avoid it at all costs (Wylie and Heath 2013).

In the 1960s and 1970s, people openly joked about minority groups and used toxic stigmas against autistic people; therefore, older people who have ASD are likely to have internalised these stigmas, which can cause depression and low self-esteem, and which means that many of us have difficulty accepting our condition completely.

'Remember, if you have gone through your entire life thinking you are different from others, and have been treated as an outcast or "less than", it is likely that you have partially internalised these ideas', says Debra Moore (correspondence, 5 January 2013). This means that our subconscious minds have at least partially accepted other people's negative beliefs about us.

There are many other reasons why we have been slow to accept our mental condition. For example, not many employers choose to recruit disabled people, and few people want a relationship with an alien. Our condition is essentially hidden, so it is commonly misdiagnosed, and even autistic people who have a formal diagnosis by a respected psychiatrist may still be doubted by family and friends. Also, many older autistic people are probably unable to discuss disability issues with parents or other relatives because those relatives may be deceased. Even when parents are alive, they may not feel comfortable having contact with their autistic son or daughter.

Finally, if there is any resistance to acceptance of a commonly misunderstood neurological condition, it follows that it would require a massive trauma to break the self-image of normalcy. A stable and sustainable economy and healthy mind, coupled with passion for special interests and social support, are our most effective panaceas.

My process of self-identification lasted over six years. I received various hints and clues from several people, but I chose not to listen to them because I could not accept myself as a disabled or otherwise 'broken being'. I had to lose all of my money and my business before I finally accepted that I am autistic.

Reaching the tipping point of self-identification

The tipping point is the event which causes self-awareness of our ASD condition, and from this point onwards our inner truth is inescapable. An example of a tipping point is a suggestion by our relationship partner that we may be autistic. The tipping point is the 'point of no return', after which our life will never be the same again.

Tony Attwood says that the two key pathways for diagnosis of adults who have ASD are:

- accidentally reading or hearing about ASD in the media and thinking, *Yes, that is me!*

- screening of other family members for ASD after a child is identified as having ASD.

Michael John Carley describes a typical scenario of how older people are initially identified as having ASD: 'Sally works on a farm and one day she reads a magazine article about autism spectrum disorder; then suddenly she gets the insight: "Hey, that's bachelor Uncle Fred!"' (Michael John Carley, interview, 16 November 2012).

The moment of Michael John Carley's self-identification

Michael John Carley's tipping point of self-identification happened shortly after his son's diagnosis. Michael vividly remembers the moment when he realised that he had ASD. He was taking a surfing holiday in Cabo, Mexico, and one evening, against his nature, he visited a nightclub. Michael's book, *Asperger's from the Inside Out: A Supportive and Practical Guide for Anyone with Asperger's Syndrome*, describes this moment: 'As the doors opened, I was jolted by the sudden acceleration of volume, and by the sight of hundreds of people, mostly young, swaying, gyrating, sweating, and drinking recklessly on multiple floors' (Carley 2008, Introduction).

It was during this moment of sensory overload in the Cabo nightclub that Michael realised with absolute certainty that he had AS. The visual freeze-frame of hundreds of twenty- and thirty-something party revellers, all moving to pulsating bass tones, is etched on his brain. This milestone was a turning point in Michael's life, and within a month he had received a formal medical diagnosis of his AS condition.

That 'eureka moment' in Cabo was essentially exciting for Michael because he knew that he was on to something big. Already an avid reader, he threw himself wholeheartedly into researching his new AS identity. Later, after starting GRASP, he would listen to hundreds of unique stories of other people diagnosed relatively late in their lives. (Michael John Carley, interview, 16 November 2012)

The tipping point represents the beginning of identity alignment, which either causes crisis or relief in the individual's mind. This experience varies according to our circumstances and beliefs. During an identity crisis, we grieve for the loss of our previous self-identity while we develop our new self-image. For example, our previous self-identity may be that of a normal, albeit eccentric, intelligent person, whereas our new identity is that of an autistic individual who thinks and acts differently, but in a predictable manner.

The healing process – from the tipping point until ultimate self-acceptance – may take weeks, months or years depending upon the support and resources available to us during this period. A period of depression is inevitable for many newly diagnosed Aspergic adults. During this stage of inner transformation, emotional support, coaching, mentoring, counselling and tender loving care are all-important.

Researching ASD and reaching self-discovery

Research leading to self-discovery is the positive and fulfilling part of the identity-alignment process. Many autistic people are naturally inquisitive – particularly about ourselves; however, be aware that there is a lot of misinformation, especially on the Internet, so *be discerning about your reference sources.*

Be wary of any articles about miracle cures for autism (because they don't exist on this planet) or any information source that focuses only on the negative symptoms of ASD. Also, despite solid evidence that autism is primarily inherited genetically, there are several misleading research studies that claim that vaccinations and other substances are the real cause of autism.

Most adults who are diagnosed as having ASD late in life take the Autism Quotient (AQ) test online (see Appendix) and later apply for a pre-diagnostic assessment or a formal diagnosis. Other self-identification sources include magazine articles, documentaries, relevant websites, posters, conversations with friends or family, and television or radio programmes. Naturally, the best way forward is to secure the support of a trusted full-time autism practitioner, such as Sara Heath of AutonomyPlus+.

Several authors on autism, including Dawn Prince-Hughes, Liane Holliday Willey and Michael John Carley, recommend maintaining a post-diagnosis journal. Michael John Carley recorded his transformational experiences in a private diary for four and a half months, noting all the changes he went through and the important insights he experienced along the way (Carley 2008).

Writing is therapeutic, so maintaining a personal development journal during the crisis is self-affirming and enjoyable. The contents of your diary may even be suitable for a blog or a book in the future.

Receiving a pre-diagnostic assessment and diagnosis of ASD

It is generally more difficult and expensive to provide a diagnosis for adults than for children. This is particularly relevant when we have no contact with parents or other relatives because there is less evidence available to confirm the genetic path of autism in the family. The revised diagnostic criteria for ASD under *DSM-5* (APA 2013) require the diagnostician to review the patient's developmental history, so some adults may be unable to provide adequate evidence.

Also, Michael John Carley says that many adults who are assessed later in life for ASD may – through prolonged pain and struggle – have learned to overcome some of the 'differences' that are listed on the diagnostic clinician's checklist. For example, some autistic people actively learn to look at other people directly in the eye, perhaps after critical comments from peers or family members; however, despite attempts to look at people directly in the eye, many of us may still appear somehow detached, as if there is no real optical contact.

Chapter 3 examines the assessment and diagnosis of ASD in more detail, but briefly, there are potentially three different stages to this part of the VLDASD experience: self-identification (via private research), pre-diagnostic assessment by an autism professional and formal diagnosis by a qualified psychiatrist or psychologist.

Ultimately, the process of diagnosis validates our personality condition by providing us with an appropriate label (e.g. ASD); however, it should be borne in mind that, while this brings peace of mind, if we take the private health care route, unless the diagnosis is used as a basis for disability allowance, or other financial support, we may never get our money back. Also, because it's just an 'opinion' based on *DSM* criteria that can and do change, the given label may also change in future. Moreover, many people, including friends and family, may disbelieve or doubt the diagnosis, even when provided by a highly respected autism diagnostician.

Unfortunately, most Aspergic adults who are diagnosed late in life have already developed some form of mental illness (such as depression, insomnia, anxiety and stress) or other secondary disorders due to lack of early identification and support. These additional issues can increase the chance of misdiagnosis because our personality has become increasingly complex over time; however, with a positive diagnosis another new stage begins.

'Coming out' and deciding in whom to confide

Usually adults 'come out' (or publicly express themselves authentically as autistic individuals) before we have fully accepted our condition. This is not surprising because some of us are never able to accept ourselves fully, and we tend to be involuntarily transparent and truthful.

Some adults with ASD tell everyone about their condition (family, friends, actual or potential relationship partner, employers), others tell no one, while the rest of us are discerning about in whom we confide. Unfortunately, impaired cognitive empathy (or theory of mind) is a common characteristic of autistic people, so we have difficulty knowing who to trust. Experiences that we may have during the coming-out process are discussed in more detail in Chapter 6.

Finding self-acceptance through enhanced understanding

Self-acceptance is the key to well-being after identity alignment. Of course, empathetic friends, family and relationship partner, as well as an opportunity to be productive in a meaningful pastime that adds value to society, facilitates self-acceptance. Unfortunately, not many of us have the support and resources available – including coaching, mentoring, counselling, support groups, mental health consultations and like-minded 'inclusive' business partners – to enable a smooth transition at such a late stage in life; however, through enhanced knowledge and awareness that we may experience negative emotions such as anger, depression and suicidal feelings, we can find self-acceptance.

> When this happens it does help to have someone as a guide. The guide could be a support professional, a mentor (either Aspies who accept their condition or an autism mentor) or a supportive relationship partner. The mentor needs to be fully trained about ASD or an Aspie themselves. Without such support, the person would be lost and lonely, without any sense of direction or purpose – like a ship without a rudder, buffered by the winds and the tides. An appropriate relationship partner can encourage the individual to reach self-acceptance. Psychotherapists and counsellors are trained to work with neurotypical people, not people who have ASD. Those with ASD easily spot fakes. It is not recommended to intervene with an Aspie mind without fully understanding ASD. (Tony Attwood, interview, 13 November 2013)

A useful method for attaining self-acceptance is simply to focus on positive, productive tasks and watch projects grow into successful ventures. In my case, I suggested a survey of late-diagnosed adults to Sara Heath of Autonomy, and thankfully, she agreed. About four months later, we published our first UK survey report (Wylie and Heath 2013) about the late diagnosis of ASD. This achievement boosted my confidence during my crisis.

Many older autistic people have only a handful of friends, and typically online pen pals. It is very important to seek connections with like-minded people – that means people with similar values and interests, who are honest, reliable and genuinely interested in us. It's much better to have two genuine friends than two hundred fickle acquaintances who don't care about us at all.

Good relationship connections flourish at autism support groups. The National Autistic Society provides a list of autism support groups around the UK, and some similar organisations in other countries are listed in the directory at the back of this book.

Finally, self-acceptance is stimulated by feelings of gratitude. A useful exercise is to help other autistic people (or indeed anyone who needs support), because by helping others we heal ourselves; therefore, a vital key to self-acceptance is to be aware of all of our advantages, and to make ourselves feel better by doing something creative and productive to make this world a better place.

Having a sustainable future

It is generally accepted that the happiest autistic adults work in their area of special interest. It also helps if we have children or a relationship partner, and a support worker, to provide company and guidance. The ingredients of a sustainable and happy future are a balanced economy, meaningful work, genuine friends and good health.

Autism support groups enable like-minded people to befriend each other. Autistic adults, therefore, may find good friends within the autism community; however, beware that there are not only autistic people pretending to be neurotypical, there may well be neurotypical people pretending to be autistic to access support services for disabled people.

Lastly, try to do adequate physical exercise each day, or as regularly as possible. Of course, it's difficult to motivate ourselves to run five kilometres when we are feeling tired, depressed or unwell, but there are many benefits, including improved sleep and enhanced mood. This topic is discussed in greater detail in Chapter 7.

Chapter 2

LIVING PRE-DIAGNOSIS

The purpose of this chapter is to highlight the key issues associated with being undiagnosed and with having a late diagnosis of ASD. These issues, which are caused by lack of self-understanding and inadequate support, worsen with age; so it follows that we should diagnose our condition at our earliest possible opportunity. While parts of this chapter will make for uncomfortable reading, it's important to remember that after diagnosis (or self-identification), our values change and we become more grounded and realistic about our strengths and weaknesses, and both practical and responsible. It's true to say that after our identity alignment (which follows self-identification) we embark upon a new life.

Michael Fitzgerald describes the consequences of not diagnosing ASD before 13 years of age as 'devastating'. 'The consequences include deep depression, suicidal ideas, poor school performance, academic deterioration, dropping out of school, anxiety and sometimes suicidal attempts or complete suicide' (Michael Fitzgerald, interview, 10 October 2013).

This chapter highlights many problems caused by late diagnosis of ASD. Unfortunately, there are few advantages, if any, by delaying our self-understanding; therefore, this chapter is necessarily the most negative part of the book. So, if you are already aware of the main issues caused by delayed diagnosis and intervention, you may consider proceeding to Chapter 3.

While living without self-understanding is bewildering and chaotic, it is sometimes exciting because we can be whoever we want to be in a life full of surprises and misunderstandings; however, being exposed to ignorance about autism and endemic prejudice after self-identification can be terrifying, especially if we thought we were essentially normal prior to diagnosis. Nevertheless, is it much better to live with self-understanding.

Many undiagnosed autistic adults struggle to survive on social support, and most are unable to sustain employment for prolonged periods. Typically, undiagnosed middle-aged autistic people are single, separated or divorced, with a history of many broken relationships and gaps in between truncated employment contracts. Of course, there are also some lucky autistic adults who have always had the support of their family and who are able to earn their own living and sustain meaningful relationships.

Late diagnosis of ASD without appropriate support usually leads to various forms of mental illness, including stress, depression, anxiety, insomnia and phobias. Many undiagnosed autistic adults, and many of those diagnosed late in life, contemplate suicide. Being rejected – or not fully accepted – by our parents is also a major contributing factor that undermines our self-esteem. Additionally, many autistic people are penalised in the employment marketplace and by society for being different. Ironically, many autistic people need more security and stability than neurotypical people do, yet most people on the spectrum receive much less financial and emotional support than the norm. Moreover, it can be extremely humiliating being dismissed as an idiot by normal people who may be less intelligent than us. What, we may ask ourselves, is the advantage of being 'gifted' if we are unable to apply these gifts and most people are not even aware of their existence? In my view, autistic people represent an undervalued section of society and, moreover, many of us lack much-needed emotional and financial support.

If our condition remains undiagnosed without any support, we will inevitably develop several problems while missing out on opportunities during our potentially productive years. Discovering that we are at the bottom of our social 'caste system', like India's 'untouchables', can be a debilitating shock for late-diagnosed adults, and one of the main consequences of VLDASD is a potentially traumatic post-diagnostic crisis.

My delayed diagnosis caused me many problems, including:

- I had numerous arguments and misunderstandings inside and outside of my family, which, over time, took their toll on my self-esteem.

- Lack of awareness of my vulnerability to stress and anxiety caused these issues to grow instead of being treated.

- I was unfairly 'constructively dismissed' by a top-four firm of accountants for another person's negligence. I lost my job because I was unaware that I had ASD and did not know my legal rights. If I had received an early diagnosis, maybe I could have accessed support from an 'inclusive' employer.

- I attracted many inappropriate friends and relationship partners over the years because I lacked cognitive empathy (without being aware of it) and I did not realise that autistic people are often severely mistreated.

- Some predatory women used me for their own selfish purposes, but without proper self-understanding, I was unable to protect myself against them.

- In 2003, I had to move to Thailand as a 'refugee' because I could not survive in the UK – even as a chartered accountant with an MBA – as I had no support and I seemed to be discriminated against in the job market.

- I chose inappropriate careers because I did not know myself properly.

- I engaged in many cross-cultural relationships due to prejudice from neurotypical British society, but this strategy tended to compound misunderstandings.

- I experienced 'identity diffusion' during my search to identify my true self, so I tried out many unsuitable 'careers'.

- I spent my savings trying to fathom myself out using therapies, natural treatments and 'wonder cures'… So I was seeking cures for a condition that cannot ever be cured! If I had understood my condition earlier I would have saved a lot of money.

- I developed depression and other mental health problems due to the delay in my diagnosis.

- I experienced a mental breakdown when I finally realised that I have ASD at the age of 51. This nearly cost me my life because I did not receive the support I needed. If I had been diagnosed during childhood, I would not have experienced a mental breakdown.

In the remainder of this chapter we will look in more detail at the key consequences of a very late diagnosis of ASD. I hope that after reading this you will realise that delaying the diagnosis can be lethal and it also potentially robs us of opportunities that arise during what should be 'productive' years.

Potentially traumatic post-self-identification crisis

Very late diagnosis of ASD can be potentially dangerous unless the individual has a strong support network following diagnosis. However, the majority of autistic adults are single and living alone without supportive family connections.

> I believe that the ASD population of late-diagnosed people can be split into two – those who already knew that they have ASD, and those for whom it comes as a surprise. The two populations are likely to have very different needs. *If* supported appropriately, the diagnosis should prove to be useful – but this is a very big 'if'. Post-diagnostic support is often either non-existent or inadequate, and yet it is absolutely crucial in terms of allowing the individual to best understand who they are, as opposed to who they thought they were – and, then, what to do about it. Many late-diagnosed individuals will go through their own grieving process, and they need highly specialised support in doing so – such support is often unavailable to the individual. Without appropriate support the consequences are potentially dire; misinformation is likely to be collated by the individual which has the potential to impact severely on the mental health of the individual. In contrast, appropriate specialised support

specific to the needs of the individual can have extremely beneficial effects. (Luke Beardon, correspondence, 31 January 2013)

Self-identification of ASD usually provides us with an explanation for many of our failures and misunderstandings, while many of our dreams disintegrate into a billion fractals. If we have been unable to make a success of our life by the age of 50 or 60, what chance, we may well ask, do we have of turning our life around after our late diagnosis? Have we outwitted ourselves by understanding ourselves too late?

It is very difficult for the late-diagnosed Aspie *not* to feel 'broken' following self-identification, especially if we don't have access to significant emotional, financial and therapeutic support. The things that keep older people living in a healthy, happy state are their home, financial security and family relationships; however, many late-diagnosed adults lack these essentials.

Moreover, without appropriate post-diagnostic support during the identity alignment stage, our mental health is likely to deteriorate. During identity alignment, we need accurate information about our condition as well as emotional support, otherwise we may feel overwhelmed by confusion and loneliness. Unfortunately, society generally takes the view that adults have been given sufficient time to get their life in order, so if we identify our mental condition during or after midlife, we may feel that we never had a genuine chance in life. In order to understand the feelings and situations that might arise due to a late diagnosis, the following sections highlight the key issues associated with late diagnosis.

Lack of support

Seeking support can be challenging enough when we know what we need support for, but successfully accessing meaningful support is highly unlikely if we don't know why we need support or what type of support we need.

There seems to be a far better understanding of autism in children's services, so getting a diagnosis tends to be easier at an early age. Funding is extremely poor in adult services, as are referral pathways and diagnostic processes in the main. The best supports for late-diagnosed autistic people are having a supportive partner, a meaningful occupation and a good understanding (and acceptance) of self. (Luke Beardon, correspondence, 31 January 2013)

Statistics show that the overriding majority of autistic adults live alone without any form of employment. In our survey, 75 per cent of the respondents lived on a pension or disability benefits, while just 15 per cent were in paid employment (Wylie and Heath 2013, pp.12–13).

Mental ill health

Most adults who are diagnosed with ASD late in life experience secondary mental health problems before and after diagnosis. Sara Heath refers to 'yo-yo-like mood swings' – similar to bipolar disorder – as being prevalent among the population of autistic adults. The pre-diagnostic mental health issues are caused mainly by environmental factors (such as bullying, prejudice, lack of social opportunities and being misunderstood) and the confusion that goes with not understanding our self. The diagnosis itself may exacerbate existing mental health issues or it may come as a positive relief, depending upon how realistic our previous self-image was and whether we have access to appropriate post-diagnostic support and accurate information about ASD.

Many adults diagnosed late in life experience diagnosis positively, with relief. At last, after many years of groping for answers to our problems, we eventually discover the real reason for our suffering. This diagnosis explains why we think and behave differently, and why we were unable to excel in a neurotypical-dominated world that is still ignorant to, and consequently intolerant of, the reality of neurodiversity. Without the self-knowledge and accompanying support associated with diagnosis, it would be unusual for an autistic adult to live successfully and harmoniously; therefore, most of us experienced mental health issues *before* our diagnosis, and many of us feel better mentally afterwards.

The three most commonly accepted co-occurring mental health issues are depression, pathological anxiety states and obsessive–compulsive disorder (OCD). The latter issue is an interesting one, as it is very often difficult for the clinician to ascertain whether it is actually OCD or a coping mechanism derived from anxiety. If it is indeed a coping mechanism, then trying to reduce it can actually be harmful. Unfortunately, in my experience, this is exactly what tends to happen. (Luke Beardon, correspondence, 31 January 2013)

The graph in Figure 2.1 is adapted from our survey (Wylie and Heath 2013) and shows, interestingly, that every respondent experienced some form of mental health issue, including anxiety.

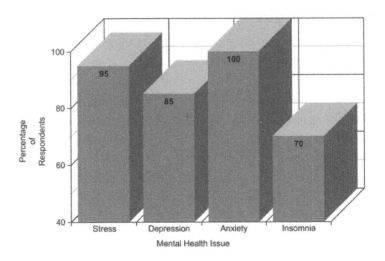

Figure 2.1 Mental ill health

Figure 2.1 also indicates that 70 per cent of survey respondents experienced insomnia. According to the Asperger's Association of New England (AANE), other research studies have found that 73 per cent of children with ASD experience sleep problems (Goldberg and Berkman 2013), so the prevalence of insomnia may not change much with age.

I don't particularly wonder what I would be like if I didn't have Asperger's syndrome. But I do wonder what I would be like with just ASD, but without being further disabled by depression, anxiety, especially social anxiety, low self-confidence and serious self-image problems. (Beardon 2011, p.144)

In *The Complete Guide to Asperger's Syndrome*, Tony Attwood states:

Children and adults with ASD may have levels of anxiety, sadness or anger that indicate a secondary mood disorder. There may also be problems expressing the degree of love and affection expected by others. Fortunately, we now have successful psychological treatment programs to help manage and express emotions. (Attwood 2006, Chapter 6)

Unfortunately, a common issue among older autistic individuals is distrust of the medical profession, especially psychiatrists and psychiatric hospitals.

'The common perception of mental health problems (i.e., the image that springs to mind when the subject is mentioned) is typically that of wild-haired 'crazies' shouting at invisible people, straitjackets, rubber-walled cells and electro-shock therapy – or is that just me?' asks Neil Shepherd. (Beardon 2011, p.99)

Online mental health screening tests are available at the American Psychiatric Association's (APA) website. These online interactive tests are short (typically with just 10 to 15 questions), so the results are available within a minute or so, and they are free of charge. The APA has three tests that may be useful for screening mental health issues:

- Depression Screening Test (http://allpsych.com/tests/diagnostic/depression.html)

- Anxiety Screening Test (http://allpsych.com/tests/diagnostic/anxiety.html)

- Stress Vulnerability Quiz (http://allpsych.com/tests/self-help/stresstest.html).

Mental exhaustion

Many late-diagnosed autistic adults experience mental exhaustion due to intense mental activity, and from trying to survive in a 'strange' world using intellect rather than instinct and intuition. Constant brainstorming about how to solve life's problems is very tiring, so whenever possible, physical relaxation is recommended during periods of exhaustion. Without understanding ourselves properly, we are at risk of exceeding our stress threshold. Prolonged intense mental activity without sufficient relaxation can cause our mind to 'crash' – just like a computer system. Sara Heath uses the 'rubber band' analogy to explain this phenomenon.

Sara Heath stretches the topic of rubber bands

The rubber band analogy is appropriate for many late-diagnosed individuals. Autistic adults are elastic and flexible up to a point: they stretch thin as rubber bands do, but if they are old and worn or stretched too thin, then they snap – mentally and often physically, too. This is severe autistic overload. This is often when, like the last straw on the camel's back, they have suffered as much as they can cope with and have a severe breakdown. But in older clients who have no diagnosis and have had so much to cope with due to a lack of understanding, this overload and meltdown is seen as mental health or psychiatric problems, so many are, or have been, sectioned and/or in hospital under a voluntary section. Many people seek alternative therapies or self-medicate to stop the overload from happening again.

Overload can seem like severe depression – switching off from the world – or, conversely, mania, such as being 'high as a kite', psychosis, delusional thinking or late-onset schizophrenia, for which the person is medicated. Medication can then cause biochemical imbalance, so people who are ill remain that way and never recover, that is, if you did not have it when you went in, you will have it when you come out! (On a full section you cannot ever refuse medication!)

When ASD rubber bands stretch, they ping – and hurt others, as we well know – but not always intentionally. If they are allowed to go back to their previous shape, they can also ping and hurt on the rebound. But they do not break. They heal after a short time and can stretch again up to a point, but constant stretching means that they will start to perish as the rubber becomes more rigid.

ASD rubber bands that have snapped are never the same again. You can tie a knot in them and they will work, but they will be smaller and will never stretch as thin again, and then there is not a lot you can do with them. (Heath, correspondence, 1 September 2013)

Comorbidity

The chance of an adult experiencing other personality disorders increases with the delay in the ASD diagnosis. In Luke Beardon's experience, many autistic individuals are also dyspraxic or dyslexic, and have sensory issues (correspondence, 31 January 2013). Other common disorders that can coexist with ASD include bipolar disorder, schizophrenia, paranoia, attention deficit hyperactivity disorder (ADHD), obsessive compulsive disorder (OCD), Prader-Willi syndrome and pathological demand avoidance syndrome (PDA) (see Figure 2.2).

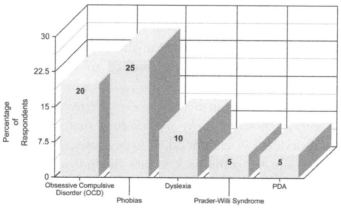

Figure 2.2 Co-morbidity and previous diagnoses

While ASD, which is usually present at birth, is incurable, attachment disorder – when the infant or mother reject the other party – typically affects children who have been neglected, abused or traumatised, but it can be treated if intervention is timely. In other words, ASD is a genetic condition, whereas attachment disorder is generally caused by adverse environmental factors during early childhood.

The characteristics of attachment disorder are similar to those of ASD, which is another reason why ASD is commonly misdiagnosed. It is therefore worth spending a few moments looking at this condition in more detail.

The child psychiatrist John Bowlby developed his 'attachment theory' at the Tavistock Clinic in London. The principle of his theory is that babies who develop a secure bond with their caregiver during the critical period of their development become healthier and more resilient later in life (Baron-Cohen 2012, p.50); however, when babies are unable to develop a strong bond with their mother – especially during their first 14 months – they will lack primordial trust and the capacity to cope with stressful situations.

Simon Baron-Cohen refers to Bowlby's concept of early secure attachment between infant and mother as an 'internal pot of gold' (Baron-Cohen 2012, p.105). The first relationship we have as a child (with mother or caregiver) acts as a template by which we understand future relationships; therefore, if our primary relationship is dysfunctional, all our future relationships are likely to follow the same pattern. Children who do not experience early secure attachment may well be destined to suffer irreversible damage.

Baron-Cohen states in his book, *Zero Degrees of Empathy: A New Theory of Human Cruelty and Kindness*, that such effects are not always evident in childhood, or even adolescence and young adulthood, but can come back to bite the individual in midlife (Baron-Cohen 2012). When a child is unable to develop the feelings of trust, security and fulfilment during the important development period, he or she will seek these things in the outside material world later in life, establishing relationships with things (e.g. drugs, status symbols and social status) instead of people (Sharamon and Baginski 1991, p.41). Jonathan Green and others are encouraging mothers and their babies to socialise and play with each other during the critical childhood development period to mitigate the effects of attachment disorder later in life (Sara Heath, correspondence, 23 March 2013).

In another study, autism researcher Peter Hobson found that children who missed out on emotionally enriching interactions with their carers during their first 18 months tend to develop the same traits as children who are born with the condition (Palmer 2006, p.110); thus, Hobson's findings show that children may inherit the traits of ASD not only genetically, but also through attachment difficulties during the critical period of infant development. The mother of Aspie Temple Grandin claims that Temple physically rejected her during infancy (Grandin 1990).

Luke Beardon believes that having attachment disorder does not increase the chances of a person having ASD, and he suspects that the prevalence of attachment disorder is the same within and outside the ASD population (correspondence, 31 January 2013).

To summarise, attachment disorder develops during childhood and manifests in a number of ways in adulthood. The traits of attachment disorder include the inability to maintain relationships, distrust, and pessimism. In essence, this disorder, as with ASD, influences how we relate to others and they to us.

Anger management issues

Diagnosis of ASD and accompanying support enables autistic individuals to guard themselves against abuse. Unfortunately, late-diagnosed autistic adults are likely to have internalised over many years the negative feelings caused by abuse, misunderstandings, betrayals and injustice, and this causes anger to build up.

In our survey, 70 per cent of the respondents claimed to have anger management issues (Wylie and Heath 2013, p.26). Again, there are many reasons why late-diagnosed autistic adults have anger issues. When society judges us as inferior, it can be difficult to resist internalising this and other negative beliefs into an anger that rails, 'How can we be inferior when we are compelled to follow our heart passionately by pursuing our special interests?' True, many autistic people are unable to participate fully in the economic sector, but often that's because we have different values and prefer to choose the dynamics into which we enter.

ASD can be a very painful affliction because many of us who have it may appear normal, so some people may disbelieve us. Most of us have above-average intelligence and we tend to be more sensitive than neurotypical people, so acts of bullying and other abuse tend to cause us more pain and suffering. It is understandable that we feel angry if, because of our very late diagnosis, we experienced, or are currently experiencing, the following:

- We were bullied, abused and exploited without understanding why this occurred.

- Our parents and other relatives always refused to discuss our health issues.

- We have poor mental health, which we could have avoided if we had been diagnosed during childhood.

- We have the skills and ability, but we find it difficult to secure and maintain an appropriate job.

- We are unable to survive in our country of origin because of lack of diagnosis or support.

- We were often misdiagnosed and given inappropriate treatment, causing further damage.

Risk of misdiagnosis

The risk of misdiagnosis increases with age, and without a diagnosis we are liable to develop poor mental health, eccentric behaviour (resulting from social isolation) and possibly other developmental disorders. So the longer we delay our diagnosis, the higher the probability that the diagnostic 'opinion' will be incorrect. In our survey, 45 per cent of respondents had originally received an incorrect diagnosis (Wylie and Heath 2013, p.20) – which usually leads to inappropriate medical treatments, causing further harm to the individual.

> Many people with undiagnosed ASD have had previous experiences with mental health counsellors or psychiatrists, and often these encounters were more frightening than helpful. You may have been given one or more psychological diagnoses over the years. These diagnoses may have been given with what seemed like complete confidence on the part of the professional, and yet you never felt that they really fit. But perhaps you told yourself they 'must know what they are talking about'. (Debra Moore, correspondence, 5 January 2013)

The main effect of misdiagnosis, apart from inappropriate medical treatment which may cause further harm to the individual, is increased confusion due to the diagnosis 'not feeling correct', which can lead to additional mental health issues and even other personality disorders.

> Many people I meet have a misdiagnosis of personality disorder or schizophrenia (I hesitate to say this is statistically the most common diagnosis, though). Many people will have psychiatric conditions diagnosed, such as clinical depression, acute anxiety or OCD; however, for many these are not psychiatric conditions but instead they result from poor understanding and support around their ASD. Many other individuals may not have any diagnoses at all, but will have accumulated various inaccurate labels, such as non-compliant, rude, arrogant, unfeeling and so forth. These labels can be as damaging as anything else.
>
> It is generally accepted – wrongly, in my opinion – that a 'medical' diagnosis by a general practitioner, paediatrician, psychiatrist or psychologist is required; however, just because the diagnostician is medically trained does not mean that he or she understands autism and ASD, nor is the converse accurate. The National Autistic Society provides a list of people who have put themselves forward as specialist diagnosticians, and many local authorities have their own multidisciplinary teams for children; however, this is much less likely for Aspergic adults. A huge issue

for Aspergic adults is their distrust of medical professionals, who very often lack a broad-enough understanding of ASD to be able to assess the individual appropriately. (Luke Beardon, correspondence, 31 January 2013)

'Some young adults are referred for a psychiatric assessment for schizophrenia and some adults who have Asperger's syndrome (ASD) may develop what appear to be signs of paranoia' (Attwood 2006). According to our survey, it is also common for autistic people to be misdiagnosed as having bipolar disorder or multiple personality disorder (aka *dissociative identity disorder*) (Wylie and Heath 2013, p.20).

In light of the above information, it is understandable that many autistic adults distrust medical professionals given the recent history of autism and the disturbing statistics concerning the prevalence of misdiagnosis among autistic adults. But whether we are awaiting a correct diagnosis or have received a late diagnosis, what are the other life issues that we may have to face?

Challenging issues for autistic people

Unemployment

Delayed diagnosis certainly causes autistic adults to have an unfair disadvantage in the workforce. Getting and keeping a job may be a problem for many autistic adults. There is probably a higher rate of ASD among the chronically unemployed. The main problems concern social or team aspects and understanding social conventions such as looking at someone for too long (Attwood 2006).

Autistic people are good systemisers and adept at solving complex problems, but unfortunately we are unable to manage people's feelings. Tony Attwood believes that autistic people:

usually have a strong desire to seek knowledge, truth and perfection with a different set of priorities than would be expected with other people. There is also a different perception of situations and sensory experiences. The overriding priority may be to solve a problem rather than satisfy the social or emotional needs of others. (Attwood and Gray 1999, p.3)

The main challenges faced by autistic people in the workplace are:

- inability to delegate and manage people (because we appear to be different)

- poor executive functioning, so project management may be challenging

- difficulty feeling comfortable in many office environments due to sensory overload, rigid procedures and rules

- difficulty respecting bosses who lack merit, integrity or management ability

- having divergent values and vision compared with those of employers, whose primary objective is to deliver maximum return on investment to their shareholders

- experiencing bullying, herd instinct and office politics, which can cause anxiety and depression

- difficulty adhering to rigid working hours during periods of mental ill health.

Low self-esteem

Inevitably, undiagnosed or late-diagnosed adults who have ASD also have low self-esteem. Such individuals often have a history of many broken relationships on all levels – from friends and family to employers and relationship partners – and eventually they tire of being misunderstood. Most autistic people are deemed wrong (while neurotypical people are assumed to be right), so it's not surprising that older undiagnosed, misdiagnosed or late-diagnosed autistic people often doubt themselves and lack confidence.

People who have low self-esteem often feel like outsiders, and for people who have ASD, this can lead to issues with authority. Autistic people think logically and often have difficulty accepting illogical conventions as well as inadequate figures of authority (whether parents, bosses or 'gatekeepers'), as exemplified by 8Ball who said:

> I suppose my troubles with authority started as a child, from asking questions when I wasn't supposed to, and asking further questions when given unsatisfactory answers, to being accused of lying when I was telling the truth – probably due to the 'eye contact' thing. (8Ball, cited in Beardon 2011, p.63)

8Ball believes that when people answer a reasonable question with 'it just is' or similar, they are appealing to their own authority (Beardon 2011, p.63). They probably don't know why certain rules exist, and they have probably never questioned them. It can be very frustrating for relatively intelligent – albeit quirky – people to be treated as idiots by authority figures who refuse to question the very rules that they enforce. Very often we ask logical questions innocently, genuinely trying and wanting to understand the relationship between 'things'.

Abandonment

Undiagnosed autistic adults have a much higher chance of being rejected or abandoned by their parents and relatives than do diagnosed children. Parents from the older generation are typically more prejudiced against disabled people and lack empathy.

Naturally, there is much more support available for children, but older people have less flexible mindsets and therefore find change more difficult to navigate; therefore, many autistic adults live alone without a carer or relationship partner, and with minimal social contact other than with online penfriends and members of local support groups.

Isolation

Autistic individuals often have great difficulty coping with conflict. Unfortunately, owing to our lack of cognitive empathy, we often misunderstand other people, and vice versa. Misunderstandings tend to result in arguments, disagreements and conflict, which compounds mental health issues, and this may result in isolation; therefore, many people who have ASD spend more time with computers than with people. Apart from lacking cognitive empathy, there are several other reasons why autistic people struggle with relationships.

As mentioned above, many autistic adults have low self-esteem and lack assertiveness. This means that our friends or acquaintances tend to choose *us*, rather than the other way around. Lack of assertiveness means that people who have ASD find it difficult to say 'no', so we may attract manipulative people.

A universal law of attraction states that like energies attract each other, and this is true of people who have personality 'conditions'. Many autistic adults have friendships with people who have personality 'disorders' such as dyslexia, bipolar disorder, dissociation, attachment disorder and narcissistic personality disorder. Also, many of us are extremely sensitive and easily affected by the depression of other people, unless we are able to protect ourselves.

Furthermore, our generosity and naïvety make us susceptible to people with dishonourable intentions. Each time we are deceived, we retreat further inside ourselves and take less initiative to meet other people.

A consequence of spending too much time alone is increased eccentricity and social awkwardness. Eccentricity, or quirky behaviour, is a result of doing things in a unique way, usually because we spend too much time alone, without feedback from other people. An effective way for many adults with ASD to meet like-minded friends is by attending groups that support our hobbies and interests.

Parenting

Late-diagnosed Aspergic adults may have children but are not always aware of the relatively high risk of our child being autistic or otherwise disabled. Everyone has the right to have children with a consenting partner, but when making this decision it's helpful to know that your son or daughter may inherit autism genetically, or develop a learning disability or other personality disorder; therefore, a timely diagnosis of ASD is beneficial to potential parents and their children.

Michael John Carley estimates that around 40 per cent of parents who give birth to autistic children consider themselves as potentially autistic (interview, 16 November 2012), but the remaining 60 per cent may or may not understand the condition and be capable of supporting their child through it, because they prefer not to identify with ASD personally. So many autistic adults become aware of their own mental condition after having children, and paradoxically, it's often the children who wake us up to our process of self-identification.

Denial of autism by parents and other relatives is common, because the condition is usually inherited genetically and is potentially embarrassing, as it provokes stigmas. Most of Michael's family did not want him to seek a diagnosis, and some wanted him to keep the outcome a secret. Michael says, 'We have to remember that, because of the genetics involved, and because of the new interpretations of the past that will have to be explored, we are not the only ones affected by our diagnosis' (interview, 16 November 2012).

Carol-Anne gave birth to two autistic daughters and an autistic son before she was diagnosed as having ASD. One of Carol-Anne's daughters and her young son also have pathological demand avoidance. If Carol-Anne had received a diagnosis during her childhood, she could have been forewarned about the potential issues that her children would have. Nevertheless, Carol-Anne's children are happy and adequately supported (correspondence, 14 February 2013).

Early diagnosis, therefore, enables autistic individuals to make informed decisions about whether to have children after considering the chances that they may inherit autism. Most people would agree that bringing up an autistic child is challenging, but what about the welfare of the child? Also, late-diagnosed adults who lack support are unlikely to be able to provide adequate support for their children.

Societal exclusion

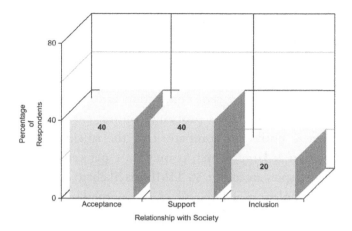

Figure 2.3 Support, acceptance and inclusion

Overall, there is irrefutable evidence that the quality of life of many autistic adults is so poor that most of us feel excluded from society. The graph in Figure 2.3 is from our survey (Wylie and Heath 2013, p.29) and shows the extent to which our respondents feel that they are part of society in terms of receiving support and acceptance and feeling included.

Self-harm and risk of suicide

It's clear from Figure 2.3 that the majority of late-diagnosed adults do not feel included by society. In fact, 80 per cent of respondents in our survey said they do not feel included in society. The same percentage stated that they think about suicide, and some reported that they contemplate it daily (Wylie and Heath 2013, p.28).

Lack of inclusion may well be a contributory factor that drives us to contemplate taking our life, which is often presaged by self-harming. Luke Beardon confirms that a significant proportion of those people seeking a late diagnosis have had self-harm issues at some point in their lives (correspondence, 31 January 2013). Among the respondents to our survey, 50 per cent had engaged in self-harm (including self-mutilation, self-poisoning and other forms of self-injury) (Wylie and Heath 2013, p.28).

> According to the National Institute of Mental Health, between 4 per cent and 12 per cent of suicidal people actually kill themselves. If we take our lowest estimate that 8 per cent of Aspies have considered suicide and multiply that by the lower estimate of [a] 4 per cent completion rate, then we find that 0.32 per cent of Aspies probably commit suicide. Not a big number – until you compare it to the suicide rate for the population at large, which is only 0.01 per cent. That would indicate Aspies are about 30 TIMES as likely to commit suicide as the population at large. (I know my methods here are not scientifically supportable and my mathematics are ghetto, but I think we've at least made our point.) (Anon, www.wrongplanet. net 2013)

The prevalence of suicidal thinking among autistic people is partially due to our logical minds. We may ask ourselves, 'What is the point in living if we cannot do what we want or gain acceptance by family or society?' Alternatively, we may ask, 'What is the point of putting up with such a poor quality of life because of society's prejudice towards us?'

Let's end this chapter by asking autism expert Tony Attwood the critical question, 'What are the chances of an undiagnosed autistic person being successful (without self-knowledge of his or her neurological condition)?'

> The odds are stacked against undiagnosed adults because they make unwise decisions based on their weaknesses rather than strengths. If they have been successful, it likely has been through a supportive relationship partner who gives them the moral and emotional support, guidance and confidence they need.
>
> Another related question is how can autistic adults cope with the ignorance and prejudice of other people towards people who are different? Some people are kind and supportive, whereas others can become predatory. So the problem is not limited to coping with ASD; the greater problem is coping

with other people. People with ASD don't suffer from their neurological condition, but they do suffer from the attitude and ignorance of other people. In my clinic I refer to 'the psychology of predators'. The person with ASD cannot have closure of their concerns until they understand why they are victimised, passed over for jobs, fail job interviews and not successful in their relationships. I explain the psychology and motivation of other people; otherwise, there tends to be either negative self-evaluation or anger towards the thoughts and actions of other people. Both ways are not constructive ways of dealing with the situation. Autistic adults can defuse their anger through accessing knowledge and appropriate information. I describe ASD as a different culture, so autistic people need a translator between the two different cultures. It's not so easy for autistic people to avoid predators because they are literally everywhere, whether in the office or at the church. These predators have an ability to identify relatively vulnerable targets. (Tony Attwood, interview, 24 October 2013)

Chapter 3

PRE-ASSESSMENT
AND DIAGNOSIS

Diagnosis is the key to self-understanding, so there is potential for a new life after self-identification. How can we expect other people to understand us when we do not know ourselves? Common diagnostic starting points for many late-diagnosed autistic individuals include magazine articles, television programmes or feedback from our relationship partner or other family member. The diagnostic journey may be long and confusing, and multiple clues may be necessary before we become fully aware of our condition.

There are potentially three stages of assessment for ASD, which are self-assessment, third-party pre-diagnostic assessment by an autism support professional, and formal diagnosis by a psychiatrist or clinical psychologist. Each of these three stages of assessment is covered in this chapter.

Many people who have ASD want a formal diagnosis, which can often help when claiming any governmental support services or living allowances. A formal diagnosis is also helpful as strong evidence to show friends and relatives who doubt our condition. Another major benefit of having a formal diagnosis is that the report confirms the *underlying condition* of ASD, which after decades of ignorance may be buried under other related forms of mental illness (such as stress, anxiety disorder, depression, multiple personality disorder and disassociation). The risk of misdiagnosis increases with the age of the undiagnosed individual. For example,

Michael Fitzgerald says that it is easy to misdiagnose autistic adults as having schizophrenia (Fitzgerald 2006).

Most, if not all, autism and mental health professionals claim that diagnosis of ASD is advantageous because it enables us to be aware of our strengths and weaknesses. This vital information also explains why we have always been treated differently. The recently diagnosed autistic adult may also gain access to a range of support services that include coaching, mentoring, counselling and support groups; however, despite the obvious benefits of diagnosis, the diagnosed autistic individual may experience a crisis that involves a period of depression.

Many of the respondents in our UK autism survey stated that they were relieved after receiving a positive diagnosis; however, some respondents said they were shocked by the news, although they had suspected it (Wylie and Heath 2013).

Overall, diagnosis is positively transformational, but there are some disadvantages which were introduced in Chapter 2 and of which we need to remain aware. For example, many autistic people distrust psychiatrists and medical doctors, perhaps because we have heard horror stories about abuse in psychiatric wards, or we have been misdiagnosed previously. Undiagnosed adults often have low self-esteem, other mental health issues and possibly other personality disorders resulting from lack of support. These additional issues increase the risk of misdiagnosis significantly.

Another complication for late-diagnosed adults is that we may have spent decades pretending to be normal, so observation-based diagnostic techniques may fail if we successfully managed to hide our autistic traits. For example, 'small talk' is a social survival skill that we can develop with practice, and eye contact, too, is learned behaviour.

Older people tend to be more influenced by the toxic stigmas associated with personality disorders, so many of us may resist acceptance of our condition. Also, the recently diagnosed adult may face a challenge in gaining acceptance of the condition by family and friends; after all, ASD is primarily inherited genetically, and most older people are understandably vehemently against attaching the ASD label to themselves.

Sadly, many adults go to their graves without having known about their hidden intellectual condition. Moreover, despite the UK Autism Act 2009, most primary care trusts do not know how many diagnosed autistic adults are in their region, so they would definitely not have relevant statistics for undiagnosed adults.

All diagnoses or assessments related to ASD are ultimately just opinions, even if *expert* opinions; in other words, they are subjective. One psychiatrist may have the opinion that Asperger syndrome (ASD) is a correct diagnosis, but another mental health practitioner may subsequently contradict that opinion. The diagnosis of ASD is so subjective because of the diverse nature of the condition; the symptoms presented in one autistic individual may be different from those in other individuals. For example, not all people who have ASD are unable to make direct eye contact with others, which is a criterion typically assessed by psychiatrists.

Surprisingly, there are still no biological tests for autism, so diagnostic techniques simply involve observation of the subject's behaviour. Over the past decade, researchers have dismissed possible associations between ASD and unloving 'refrigerator parents', and the combined measles, mumps and rubella vaccination; however, the Autism Research Centre at the University of Cambridge has evidence that mothers of autistic babies have excessive amounts of testosterone in their womb prior to giving birth (Baron-Cohen 2012). Moreover, research at the King's College Institute of Psychiatry has revealed that a 15-minute magnetic resonance imaging brain scan can identify ASD with 90 per cent accuracy (Wellyn 2012); therefore, biological testing for autism may be available to the lay public in the near future.

It is important that we remain completely open and truthful during our assessments and diagnoses, because erroneous answers may invalidate our diagnosis and lead to other health issues. It also pays to be thorough in our personal enquiry by collecting as much reliable data as possible about our developmental history. This research may include a review of our school reports, essays and drawings, family photographs and journals. Do not hide any details because of fear of embarrassment; conversely, provide as much accurate information about your life as possible to maximise your chances of an accurate diagnosis, which is your passport to a new life with sufficient and appropriate support.

Another diagnostic pathway is referral by an alcohol agency or drug addiction support services. Sarah Hendrickx describes typical diagnostic pathways for late-diagnosed individuals.

> Alcoholism and drug use tend to mask Asperger syndrome. It may not be until the point that the alcohol makes you ill or nearly dead that you come into contact with mental health services, and then somebody may diagnose you as being on the autistic spectrum.
>
> Alcohol makes you more flexible. It's a social uninhibitor that makes the world less sharp. You don't notice as much. You can wander around in your own little bubble. That certainly was the case for lots of people I spoke to when researching my book.
>
> I think a lot of alcoholics and drug users with Asperger syndrome may not yet have got a diagnosis. They're just drinking. Their drinking means they don't need a diagnosis yet. But there might come a point in their life in their forties or fifties when the alcohol becomes a bigger problem. The number of Aspies who use alcohol to self-medicate is unknown because they are undiagnosed and hidden behind the alcohol. Every now and then I get a call from some alcohol agency saying, 'We've got this person we think has Asperger syndrome.' Standard treatment isn't working because there is an assumption that the alcoholism is the primary problem – alcohol addiction – whereas I believe that it's the Asperger syndrome that's the primary problem and the alcohol is actually the cure, solution or strategy. If you try to treat them with alcohol rehab before treating the primary condition (ASD), you're going to fail because as soon as you take away the cure (alcohol), the Aspie will go back into extreme anxiety, so they will need to drink

again. So we need to put something else in place before we take away the alcohol.

Alcohol and mental health are very closely linked, so anxiety disorders and alcoholism are also closely connected. Asperger syndrome is really only one or two steps away from that in terms of experiencing anxiety. I've said for many years that I'm a much better person with about half a pint of cider in me at all times. When I have a patch with just about that much alcohol inside – no more, no less – I'm a much easier going, happier, calmer person.

After a friend of mine stopped drinking, he had to make his life smaller because he couldn't maintain mortgage, job, wife and other commitments without the alcohol. The alcohol was enabling all of that to be possible. It was making him flexible. It was making him more tolerant. It was making him more capable. When the alcohol went, the anxiety – or whatever it is that characterises Asperger syndrome – was raw. He had to change where he lived. He had to change his job. He just worked part time. He just had to shrink the world because his capacity had shrunk. It wasn't a case of just stopping the alcohol. Something else has got to give as well because the alcohol potentially is fulfilling some function for you. Some lifestyle change has to come with that.

I think it's a neurotypical expectation that you're not going to be anxious and you're not going to be depressed. If you see the world the way an Aspie sees it, you are going to be anxious and depressed because you don't fit in. Everything is confusing and overwhelming. I think it's almost given that you will be anxious and depressed, so we work from that point onwards rather than just trying to numb it with some kind of medication. This view that anxiety is an intrinsic part of the experience of life with an ASD is widely held in the autism field. I guess you could say that with neurotypical people, anxiety and depression are two irrational mental health problems. For people with Asperger syndrome, it's a perfectly rational explanation and response because you're left out and you don't understand it.

It's fair game that I'm going to feel anxious. I'm scared of most people because I don't know what they're going to do next. That's perfectly reasonable to me. I don't want medication for that. That's not going to help. If I'm medicated, I still can't read anybody. It's not going to solve the problem. The quality of the anxiety or depression, as well as the cause of it, is an entirely different thing for Aspies than it is for neurotypical people. They want to get rid of the mental health issues without healing the underlying cause, and of course it doesn't work. (Sarah Hendrickx, interview, 20 November 2013)

Self-assessment

Self-assessment (or self-identification) is, of course, a personal opinion which may be validated later by a clinical psychologist or psychiatrist. This stage does not involve any third-party autism professionals, psychologists or psychiatrists, so it is limited to desk research and communication with family and friends.

Genetic pathway

Since ASD is essentially a hereditary condition, research into the family's genealogy may reveal a clear genetic pathway of autism. Certain ancestors may have been eccentric or quirky, and possibly mentally ill or even hospitalised. Other typical signs of an autistic ancestor are living a solitary or reclusive life, chronic unemployment and inability to sustain marital relationships. These relatives may have above-average intelligence, intense focus on their special interests and some success in fields such as maths, writing, music and philosophy. Whether they were gifted or simply eccentric, they may have been people with undiagnosed ASD.

One of my godfathers set me on the right path towards identifying the genetic path of autism in my family with the following message:

Your grandmother's brother was a tea planter or manager in India and he would come home now and again. It was great to see him as he was very entertaining and brought a new world to us kids, but he was a bachelor and perhaps may have been 'different' – he exhibited many traits of ASD.

The main characteristics to look for among ancestors are:

- inability to hold any job for long, or chronic unemployment

- many broken relationships, including divorce and separation

- lonesome or reclusive behaviour, and undue sensitivity

- eccentric behaviour

- excessive use of alcohol and/or other drugs to self-medicate

- attendance of many schools owing to learning difficulties

- above-average intelligence with intense 'special' interests

- insomnia and the use of sleeping tablets

- a married couple sleeping in separate beds or even different bedrooms.

Tony Attwood estimates that 46 per cent of first-degree relatives of people who have ASD have a similar profile of abilities and behaviour (Attwood 2006); therefore, an analytical review of personality types in the family can reveal the genetic pathway of autism in many cases. Diagnosticians should therefore investigate the genetic pathway of ASD on a family basis, rather than individually.

Be aware that most psychiatrists, diagnosticians, psychologists and autism support professionals will not assist us in this important task of identifying the genetic pathway of our condition. I asked several practitioners to assist me in this way, but not one of them agreed to help. Why? The reason is that they are concerned about possible conflict with other family members who are unable to come to terms with their ASD condition. So although they may cite professional ethics as their reason for non-engagement, they may be trying to protect themselves.

Childhood development issues

During infancy autistic children may exhibit symptoms of their condition, which may include temper tantrums, delayed motor skills, lack of coordination and introspection. It is often in retrospect that the obvious warning signs of autism become apparent, such as reluctance to play with other children or the perception that everyone apart from the child seemed to understand society's 'invisible rules'. Autistic children tend to get into trouble at both school and home without understanding why because people incorrectly assume that they are being naughty wilfully. Relatives or friends may have commented on our obsessive habits or routines, or our oddly mature speech patterns as we mimicked adults without fully understanding what we were saying.

It may have been difficult to form close emotional relationships, or conversely, the strength of an emotional attachment may have made its recipient uncomfortable. This may have led to feelings of loneliness and frustration.

Reflecting on our childhood, autistic individuals may recall times when we had unexpected meltdowns without understanding why. Perhaps someone had disturbed our much-loved routine, or we were frustrated at being unable to communicate with a friend or authority figure. We may also recall specific activities that we used to relax or to cope with uncomfortable situations. For example, we may have looked for reasons not to eat lunch with other children to prevent us from worrying about where we would sit. If you recognise any of the above experiences, further diagnostic assessment probably would be beneficial.

Some autistic people, including Temple Grandin, may also have developed attachment disorder as an infant (Grandin 1990) and, as discussed in Chapter 2, these effects can become more evident in later life.

Self-assessment tests

Whether or not, as adults with ASD, we choose to obtain a formal diagnosis, many of us have become aware of our hidden condition by reading relevant books and articles, and taking online self-assessment tests. These tests differ from the APA's tests mentioned in Chapter 2 which focus on aspects of mental health; however, before moving on to describe these useful self-assessment tests, it is necessary to have some understanding of the scientific criteria upon which most of these tests are based.

As mentioned earlier, the formal criteria for ASD are listed in the *Diagnostic and Statistical Manual of Mental Disorders*, which covers mental disorders as defined in the USA and is respected internationally. The fifth edition (*DSM-5*; APA 2013) has been available since May 2013. Information about how the manual has evolved with respect to ASD (including Asperger syndrome) is available online (see www.dsm5.org).

The APA states that anyone diagnosed under the previous edition, *DSM-IV*, with autistic disorder, Asperger disorder, childhood disintegrative disorder or the umbrella diagnosis of pervasive developmental disorder, should meet the criteria for ASD or another disorder listed in *DSM-5* (APA 2013). The APA therefore has eliminated Asperger syndrome and the other three disorders, establishing instead a single umbrella disorder called 'autism spectrum disorder' (ASD) in *DSM-5*.

This wider diagnostic classification has alarmed parents and carers of people at both ends of the autism spectrum. People who were previously diagnosed as having Asperger syndrome have milder autistic traits than people who have classic autism, yet now they are placed in the same category. On the other hand, parents and carers of severely impaired autistic people are concerned that such people will receive less support than before because the new categorisation includes high-functioning autistic people who require less support.

The APA changed the diagnostic criteria for autism to reduce the incidence of misdiagnosis and recognise that autism is defined by a set of characteristics across a spectrum from mild to severe impairment of social skills and communication. Part of the revised diagnostic procedure is to grade the severity of autistic traits from 'mild' to 'severe'. A benefit of the new diagnostic system is that diagnosticians are required to consider the individual's developmental history instead of just focusing on behavioural observation as before. Also, it is not necessary for the individual to have experienced any delay in linguistic ability for the new ASD diagnosis; however, this diagnostic approach is more challenging for adults who may have learned to hide their autistic traits (such as avoidance of eye contact), and they may not have access to family members who could verify their childhood developmental history.

Some autism advocacy organisations raised concerns that people already diagnosed with Asperger syndrome under *DSM-IV* might not meet the revised criteria for ASD in *DSM-5*; however, a study published in the *Journal of the American Academy of Child and Adolescent Psychiatry* in April 2012 reported that 60.6 per cent of cases with a diagnosed ASD (including Asperger syndrome) under *DSM-IV* met the *DSM-5* diagnostic criteria for ASD. Some researchers estimate that up to 75 per cent of previously diagnosed people with Asperger syndrome will not meet the new diagnostic criteria for ASD; therefore, many previously diagnosed autistic adults face the risk that they will not qualify for the new ASD diagnosis, so some people will lose their entitlement to disability benefits and health services.

The other major authority on personality 'disorders' is the *International Classification of Diseases and Related Health Problems* (10th edition) or *ICD-10* (World Health Organization 2012). The *ICD-10* classification of ASD is similar to that covered in *DSM-5* (with a focus on negative traits).

There are three categories of criteria that an individual must meet in order to be diagnosed with ASD. The categories are listed below along with the typical traits, which may indicate whether the individual needs further assessment:

1. **Persistent deficits in social communication and social interaction across contexts, not accounted for by general developmental delays:**

   - lack of friends and social life
   - friends often much older or younger

- mumbling and not completing sentences
- issues with social rules (such as staring at other people)
- inability to understand jokes and the benefit of 'small talk'
- introverted (shy) and socially awkward
- inability to understand other people's thoughts and feelings
- uncomfortable in large crowds and noisy places
- detached and emotionally inexpressive.

2. **Restricted, repetitive patterns of behaviour, interests or activities:**

- obsession with 'special interests'
- collecting objects (such as stamps and coins)
- attachment to routines and rituals
- ability to focus on a single task for long periods
- eccentric or unorthodox behaviour
- non-conformist and distrusting of authority
- difficulty following illogical conventions
- attracted to foreign cultures
- affinity with nature and animals
- support for victims of injustice, underdogs and scapegoats.

3. **Restricted, repetitive patterns of behaviour, interests or activities:**

- inappropriate emotional responses
- victimised or bullied at school, work and home
- overthinking and constant logical analysis
- spending much time alone
- strange laugh or cackle
- inability to make direct eye contact when talking

- highly sensitive to light, sound, taste, smell and touch

- uncoordinated and clumsy with poor posture

- difficulty coping with change

- adept at abstract thinking

- ability to process data sets logically and notice patterns or trends

- truthful, naïve and often gullible

- slow mental processing and vulnerable to mental exhaustion

- intellectual and ungrounded rather than intuitive and instinctive

- problems with anxiety and sleeping

- visual memory.

Table 3.1 Online tests

Name of Test	Website Link
Adult Asperger Assessment	http://autismresearchcentre.com/arc_tests
AQ (Autism Quotient)	http://autismresearchcentre.com/arc_tests www.wired.com/wired/archive/9.12/aqtest.html
Aspie Quiz	http://rdos.net/eng/Aspie-quiz.php
EQ (Empathy Quotient)	http://autismresearchcentre.com/arc_tests
Enneagram	http://similarminds.com/test.html
Faux Pas Recognition	http://autismresearchcentre.com/arc_tests
Giftedness Test	www.gifteddevelopment.com/ADJ/scale.htm
Myers Briggs Personality Test	www.myersbriggs.org
Reading the Mind in the Eyes Test	http://autismresearchcentre.com/arc_tests
SQ (Systemising Quotient)	http://autismresearchcentre.com/arc_tests
Theory of Mind Test	http://autismresearchcentre.com/arc_tests

The online assessment tools discussed next draw on the above knowledge and criteria, but it must be remembered that they are for self-assessment purposes only and do not constitute a formal diagnosis. The website addresses for these tests are provided in Table 3.1.

THE AUTISM QUOTIENT TEST

One of the most popular online self-assessment tools for ASD is Simon Baron-Cohen's Autism Quotient (AQ) test. Baron-Cohen developed this test at the Autism Research Centre at Cambridge (ARC) to identify people on the autism spectrum. The AQ test covers the triad of Aspergic impairments, which are social skills, communication and potential for sensory overload. The time required to take the AQ test and calculate the score is approximately 20 minutes. The test comprises a list of 50 statements, such as 'I find social situations easy', to which you give a response by selecting one of the following four categories: 'definitely agree', 'slightly agree', 'slightly disagree' and 'definitely disagree'.

In the initial trial of the AQ test, the average score in the control group was 16.4; however, 80 per cent of those diagnosed with autism or a related disorder scored at least 32. The AQ test enables us to receive a personal assessment rather than a formal diagnosis, and many people who score over 32 and meet the diagnostic criteria for Asperger syndrome (ASD) have no difficulty functioning in their everyday lives. The AQ test is reproduced in the Appendix to this book thanks to the kind permission of its authors.

THE EMPATHY QUOTIENT TEST (ADULT VERSION)

Empathy is the glue that bonds people together, so enhanced empathy leads to stronger, more robust relationships. Also, empathy can be measured, which means that it is not necessary to use judgements ranging from 'kind' or 'generous' to 'cruel' or 'evil'.

People who are on the autism spectrum tend to lack cognitive empathy, which means that we are unable to sense other people's thoughts and feelings; however, it is important to understand that autistic people have 'affective empathy', so we tend to support people who we know are suffering. Narcissists and psychopaths, on the other hand, lack affective empathy, so they tend to enjoy watching their vulnerable victims suffer (Baron-Cohen 2012).

Simon Baron-Cohen created the Empathy Quotient (EQ) test in 1998 to identify people with low empathy. The EQ test, which comprises a list of 40 statements, requires us to select one of four categories to describe how strongly we agree or disagree with each statement.

There is a straightforward method to calculate our EQ score, which takes about ten minutes (see Table 3.1). Any score below 32 is considered low, and the majority of people who have high-functioning autism (ASD) score around 20. In the average range of between 33 and 52, most women score 47 and men score about 42. Scores that are greater than 52 are above average.

As well as being available online, the adult version of the EQ test is published in the book *Zero Degrees of Empathy* (Baron-Cohen 2012). Baron-Cohen also developed a separate EQ test for children which consists of 27 statements related to the child's behaviour (Auyeung *et al.* 2009). There are separate EQ tests for children and adults because assessment of low empathy among adults is slightly more difficult than it is with children, because many adults learned to modify their quirky behaviour to fit into society better. Also, it may be difficult for adults to collect vital clues related to childhood development.

THE FAUX PAS RECOGNITION TEST (ADULT VERSION)

Social awkwardness is a trait of many autistic people, so the Faux Pas Recognition test aims to measure how likely it is that a person will make faux pas (mistakes). This test was devised by Simon Baron-Cohen and Valerie E. Stone of the ARC and comprises 20 stories which involve social interactions; participants need to answer eight questions for each situation.

The first two questions identify recognition of social faux pas by asking whether anyone said anything inappropriate in the given social situation. The third question asks about the nature of the inappropriate action. The fourth question asks about the speaker's intention and motivation. The fifth question concerns the person's beliefs. The sixth question is about the person's empathy. The final two questions are control questions.

THE SYSTEMISING QUOTIENT TEST

The Systemising Quotient (SQ) test was developed by Baron-Cohen *et al.* (2003) and is a measure of a person's ability to categorise and otherwise process data logically and to notice patterns and trends. Aspergic individuals have an above-average ability to systemise information due to our ability to think logically; therefore, a higher-than-average SQ score indicates one aspect of AS; however, on average, women have lower SQ scores than men because women tend to be more intuitive.

THEORY OF MIND TEST

The Theory of Mind (TOM) test was developed by Stone, Baron-Cohen and Knight (1998) and is a measure of the ability to sense other people's thoughts, intentions, motivations and feelings. Theory of mind is also known as cognitive empathy. As explained above, a characteristic of autistic people is our inability to sense other people's thoughts and feelings, which makes us susceptible to coercion or manipulation; therefore, autistic individuals tend to have a lower TOM score than neurotypical people, and men score less than women on this test of cognitive empathy.

GIFTEDNESS TEST

Most autistic people have above-average intelligence, but some of us are exceptionally intelligent and 'gifted'. 'Giftedness' is a neurological condition, just as autism is.

Linda Kreger Silverman describes giftedness as follows:

> Gifted children and adults see the world differently because of the complexity of their thought processes and their emotional

intensity. People often say to them, 'Why do you make everything so complicated?' 'Why do you take everything so seriously?' 'Why is everything so important to you?' The gifted are 'too' everything: too sensitive, too intense, too driven, too honest, too idealistic, too moral, too perfectionist, too much for other people! Even if they try their entire lives to fit in, they still feel like misfits. The damage we do to gifted children and adults by ignoring this phenomenon is far greater than the damage we do by labeling it. Without the label for their differences, the gifted come up with their own label: 'I must be *crazy*. No one else is upset by this injustice but me.' (Silverman 1993)

Gifted people tend to be visual thinkers, so their memory is image based, as is the case for many autistic people. The traits of gifted people exemplify the characteristics of genius including curiosity, wonder, humour, playfulness and imagination. We tend to develop as 'bespectacled professors', which usually leads to social isolation and mental health issues.

Linda Kreger Silverman has assessed over 5200 children and adults since 1979, many of whom have ASD, attention deficit disorder and dyslexia. She has produced a self-diagnostic questionnaire for adults, The Giftedness Test, which is available on the Gifted Development website (see Table 3.1).

ASPIE (ASD) QUIZ

The Aspie quiz was created by Leif Ekblad to assess both the neurotypical and autistic traits of individuals. It comprises 150 questions which require categorised responses ('don't know'; 'no/never'; 'a little'; 'yes/often'). Each of the test's statements relate to talent, compulsion, social skills, communication, hunting (basic survival skills)[1] and perception.

A major benefit of this test is that the website allows us to download a detailed report in PDF format. The report provides both neurotypical and ASD scores as well as an assessment for ASD; however, please note that this test, which is free of charge

---

1   For more information on 'Aspie hunting', see http://blog.rdos.net/?p=61.

and takes about 15 minutes to complete, is not a substitute for professional diagnosis.

OTHER SELF-ASSESSMENT TESTS

Other potentially useful self-assessment tests include the Alexithymia test for emotional conditions and the Rosenberg self-esteem test. As highlighted earlier, many people who have ASD have low self-esteem due to isolation and being undervalued by family and society; therefore, low self-esteem is an associated mental health issue that arises from late diagnosis and lack of support.

Pre-diagnostic assessments

After using online self-assessment tools and receiving confirmation that we may have ASD, we are likely to want some form of third-party validation to confirm our suspicion. Many psychologists, social workers, clinicians and autism support workers who have extensive training and experience related to autism provide 'pre-diagnostic assessments' for ASD. The consultation is usually conducted face to face, but it may be done via video call. The interview typically lasts 60–90 minutes.

The pre-diagnostic assessment is an informal opinion by a third-party autism professional which is contained in a professional report. The report is often addressed, 'To whom it may concern' because many autistic people use the pre-diagnostic assessment to pass on to their doctor, clinical psychologist or psychiatrist for formal diagnosis.

Sara Heath is AutonomyPlus+'s specialist autism support worker who provides pre-diagnostic assessments from Shropshire in the UK. On the Autonomy website (www.shopshireautonomy. co.uk), Sara describes these assessments and the service she provides as follows:

> It can often be frustrating, difficult or expensive for an adult to gain a medical diagnosis of autism, Asperger's syndrome (ASD) and/or ADHD due to a lack of insight or understanding of the conditions from many health care professionals. Sara

Heath, Autonomy's Specialist Worker, can facilitate this process through her extensive experience of working with over 200 clients with Asperger's syndrome (ASD) and supporting over 50 local people through the diagnostic procedure. Sara can visit you in your own home if you wish, and will provide an in-depth, comprehensive, non-medical, pre-diagnostic assessment of autism, Asperger's syndrome (ASD), and/or ADHD with a written report for your doctor or health professional, if required, or a comprehensive personalised report of your condition if you prefer not to proceed with a medical diagnosis. Due to her extensive experience, Sara is also able to recognise the often hidden traits of ASD in women, who find it more difficult to gain a diagnosis.

There are several advantages of obtaining a pre-diagnostic assessment report:

- The report is written by a third-party autism professional.

- The assessment will facilitate formal diagnosis later, if required.

- The report may help to eliminate any self-doubt in connection with the self-assessment.

- Usually the assessment is provided at low cost, and sometimes on a donation basis.

- The specialist support worker who writes the report may also provide a range of other valuable support services for autistic people, such as social meetings, coaching, mentoring and support groups (known as post-diagnostic support services).

The questions asked by the autism professional during the pre-diagnostic assessment aim to validate the existence of the following autistic traits:

- awareness from the beginning that we are different

- evidence of impaired social skills and inability to understand social cues

- inability to maintain relationships with friends, family, and work colleagues
- detachment because people are unpredictable and confusing
- communication issues and being constantly misunderstood
- difficulty understanding body language
- use of complex formal words and verbosity
- difficulty understanding other people's jokes
- lack of social imagination and preference for non-fiction
- special interests which absorb our focus for long periods
- love of routines and rituals, and difficulty coping with change
- inability to hide our feelings (especially anger)
- potential for sensory overload (of all the five senses)
- inability to multitask
- visual-based memory and slower mental processing (may talk more slowly than most neurotypical people).

A positive pre-diagnostic assessment report for ASD facilitates the official diagnostic process, which must be carried out by a psychiatrist or a suitably qualified psychologist. This report reduces the chance of misdiagnosis and streamlines the diagnostic process.

Formal diagnosis

Even though the process of formal diagnosis is not always straightforward, obtaining a formal diagnosis of ASD can be positive in many ways. Many adults who are diagnosed late in life say that the self-knowledge helped them to understand the reasons for their difficulties and why they are more competent in some skills. Also, a diagnosis usually facilitates access to support and benefits. The diagnosis for autism spectrum disorder includes autism, ASD, pervasive developmental disorder, atypical autism and Asperger syndrome, which includes various forms of high-functioning autism.

The main advantages of getting a formal diagnosis are:

- sound validation to counter people – especially relatives – who persist in doubting our condition

- enhanced self-understanding and acceptance by other people

- access to a large volume of information on the Internet and elsewhere

- access to appropriate support to integrate into the local community and identify appropriate ways of living independently.

Usually the starting point for a formal diagnosis of autism is a referral from a doctor, usually a general practitioner (GP); however, many GPs are not knowledgeable about ASD, so it may be helpful to give the doctor an explanatory brochure about the condition, and ideally a pre-diagnostic assessment report.

When the GP is sufficiently convinced that the patient is autistic, he or she normally makes a referral to a registered psychiatrist or clinical psychologist. It is important to keep the focus of the meeting on the diagnosis of ASD, rather than any associated personality disorders.

When choosing a practitioner for your diagnosis, if you are given the option to do so, three important factors to consider are their knowledge, experience and level of empathy towards autistic people. Specialisation in autism is as important as tertiary education in autism.

If a practitioner who is genuinely empathetic towards autistic people is preferred, one way of gauging their attitude is to read their publications. For example, Simon Baron-Cohen clearly demonstrates his empathy in his writing. Be warned, however, that there are highly qualified psychiatrists and people with PhDs with limited knowledge about autism, while some others lack empathy towards people with ASD. Of course, it's best to consult a genuinely empathetic specialist diagnostician.

It's worth taking the time to find the right practitioner, not least because, as has been highlighted elsewhere in this book, it is important to remember that misdiagnosis can be extremely damaging because it can lead to inappropriate treatment and further confusion; therefore, it makes sense to consult the best possible autism practitioner to limit our chances of receiving an erroneous or misleading opinion. Also, try to obtain third-party references (or feedback) for each practitioner. You can read comments by members of specialist online forums about their experience with diagnosticians. The best people to ask are autistic individuals who have already received their positive diagnosis, so you may consider asking around at your local autism support group.

In the UK, the waiting list for the diagnosis of adults with ASD varies from county to county, but the lead time is typically 2–12 months. Most adults in the UK obtain diagnosis free of charge on the National Health Service (NHS), but some prefer to pay for a private consultation, which may cost up to £2000. In America, where the health system is entirely private, people usually pay thousands of dollars for diagnoses. The main advantages of 'going private' are that the diagnosis is likely to be made sooner and the report does not need to be filed with our medical records.

Sarah McCulloch's journey to getting a formal diagnosis for ASD

Since the 1990s, educational psychologists have been responsible for screening children with autism in the UK, but the system does not always work properly. Sarah McCulloch discovered that getting a formal diagnosis for ASD, as well as support from the NHS, is a byzantine process which varies enormously according to the applicant's postcode.

Sarah related to me that she grew up in London where an educational psychologist reported that she was dyslexic. Later, after moving to Essex, Sarah was assessed by a school educational psychologist and the report produced stated that she probably had dyspraxia (which is a type of developmental coordination disorder). Three years later, while obtaining a formal assessment for dyspraxia by an occupational therapist, it was concluded that Sarah met the criteria for semantic pragmatic disorder, a communication disorder which had only recently been defined. Sarah's behaviour and difficulty interacting with her peers was remarked upon at school and she was provided with counselling for three years, but no efforts were made to investigate further.

Sarah repeatedly sought to secure a formal diagnosis for ASD, which she clearly recognised in herself after extensive reading on the subject. Sarah asked her GP to refer her for a formal diagnosis, but the GP did not know enough about autism.

During the subsequent four years, Sarah tried to obtain a formal diagnosis of ASD with the NHS in Manchester, but without success. It became apparent that there were no psychiatrists or clinical psychologists in Manchester then who were qualified to give the diagnosis on the NHS, whereas Sheffield had an entire diagnostic unit exclusively for autistic people.

A psychiatrist suggested that the closest appropriate service was the Sheffield Asperger Service (SAS). Sarah passed on the information and application form from the SAS to her doctor, but a referral to another primary care trust required special funding. So Sarah applied for funding, but no decision was made after two years of waiting. After five years, Sarah eventually paid £600 for a private diagnosis in Sheffield and obtained a positive opinion. (Sarah McCulloch, interview, 8 January 2013)

In the UK, access to ASD diagnosis and support varies from county to county. During the last ten years, ASD support services have improved in some parts of the UK, but not in others.

Post-diagnostic assessment and support

After a formal diagnosis, many autism professionals offer what are called post-diagnostic assessments of autistic special needs for people who need to claim assistance from social services or other forms of benefit. Sara Heath of AutonomyPlus+ provides post-diagnostic assessments for autistic people who need support from local social services departments or the Department for Work and Pensions in the UK. The service may involve an assessment of an autistic person's specific needs and a social care assessment of needs. Such assessments improve the chances of autistic people being able to access appropriate support.

Post-diagnostic support includes mentoring, explaining, translating, working with families and promoting understanding of the condition for autistic people and their families, partners, employers and friends. Other post-diagnostic services include teaching new skills and supporting people to deal with their emotions, anxiety and depression.

Although autistic individuals are often underemployed due to social issues, misunderstandings, sensory overload, stress and depression, those autistic people who are able to sustain employment tend to have a more effective support network, including supportive family and friends, as well as coaching, mentoring and counselling – but remember that a *formal* diagnosis is usually a prerequisite for access to these services.

Other psychometric tests

Before summarising the benefits of diagnosis, it may be worth mentioning that there are several psychometric tests that may facilitate the process of self-identification, even if they hold no diagnostic validity on their own. Examples of such psychometric tests are the Enneagram and the Myers Briggs test.

THE ENNEAGRAM

The Enneagram offers a model of human personality based on the metaphysical studies of George Ivanovich Gurdjieff who founded the Institute for the Harmonious Development of Man in Paris in 1922. The model is depicted typographically by a circle containing an equilateral triangle and a geometric figure containing nine points. There are nine types of human personality in the Enneagram. (The word *'ennea'* means 'nine' in the Greek language.)

Many people who have ASD have either a type 5 personality (The Detached Intellectual) or a type 4 personality (The Individualist). The type 5 with 4 wing personality is The Iconoclast, whereas the type 4 with 5 wing personality is The Bohemian.

Type 5 personalities tend to have conflicting feelings about the world and tend to spend much of their time in the realm of thought. They are good at making sense of complex situations and innovating. Moreover, they often seem ungrounded because they are so detached from the real world.

MYERS BRIGGS TEST

The Myers Briggs test is used in some human resources departments to identify the personality types of job applicants. The test measures the personality characteristics according to four dyads:

- Introspection (I) vs Extroversion (E)

- Intuition (N) vs Sensing (S)

- Thinking (T) vs Feeling (F)

- Judging (J) vs Perceiving (P).

The above four pairs of personality variables can be arranged in a 4 × 4 matrix of 16 distinct personality types, as shown in Table 3.2.

Table 3.2 Myers Briggs and ASD

ISTJ	ISFJ	INFJ	The Scientist (INTJ)
ISTP	ISFP	INFP	The Thinker (INTP)
ESTP	ESFP	ENFP	ENTP
ESTJ	ESFJ	ENFJ	ENTJ

Many people who have ASD report that they have the INTJ personality of The Scientist or the INTP personality of The Thinker. The Scientist is original, independent, analytical and able to identify patterns in external events with his or her systemising skills. The INTJ personality is also sceptical and able to focus on minute details. The Thinker, on the other hand, is an original and logical thinker who values knowledge. Usually the INTP personality is quiet, reserved, detached and individualistic.

Conclusion

While such tests as those outlined above may seem confusing initially, and the three-stage process of assessment may seem rather daunting, overall, the benefits of self-identification and/or a formal diagnosis outweigh the disadvantages by far. Debra Moore cites five significant ways in which a professional diagnosis can help (correspondence, 5 January 2013):

• You will have a framework that helps you to understand your experiences.

• You can start to view yourself more realistically and positively.

• Other people in your life can understand you better.

• Diagnosis will guide suitable counselling or coaching.

• A formal diagnosis can help you qualify for academic or workplace accommodations, or informal assistance.

However, following self-identification or diagnosis, an identity crisis may follow, and in some cases it can be severe (and potentially life-threatening if the individual is desperate), and it may last anything from three weeks to three years or longer. The thought of possibly having to endure an identity crisis may seem like a very big reason not to have a diagnosis, but there are many advantages. These advantages, and the few disadvantages, are discussed in Chapter 4.

Chapter 4

THE ADVANTAGES
AND DISADVANTAGES
OF DIAGNOSIS

The overwhelming majority of autistic people who have a formal diagnosis are pleased to have their neurological condition confirmed by a professional authority. Afterwards, the individual has various choices available with regard to how they use this life-changing information. Despite the possibility of having a challenging identity alignment crisis after the diagnosis, the following advantages inevitably outweigh any disadvantages, which tend to be temporary anyway. Below are the most common advantages and disadvantages of obtaining a diagnosis.

The advantages of diagnosis
Gaining awareness of our strengths and weaknesses
Awareness of our hidden intellectual condition facilitates our access to lots of valuable information from autism practitioners and charities, relevant media and online resources, and, particularly, Internet forums. Of course, we should be discerning of our reference sources because there is so much inaccurate and misleading information out there; however, accurate information helps us to be clearer about our gifts (strengths) as well as our weaknesses.

Although there are several traits which are prevalent throughout the autistic population, each one of us is unique. We should be aware that ASD affects each individual differently. For example, not all autistic people have impaired communication skills.

Awareness of our strengths and weaknesses can save us lots of time and suffering. It's like having a handbook for our motor vehicle so we can maintain it properly for optimal functioning; or mountaineering with a compass and map, without which we could easily get lost.

Gaining access to support services

A formal diagnosis is a prerequisite for any disabled person who wants access to social welfare benefits, health care services (including mental health), autism support groups, coaching and mentoring. Without a diagnosis, most of these services would only be available privately, which may be quite expensive.

Benefiting from improved communication

Self-identification and diagnosis improves communication because we begin to see ourselves as other people do. When we understand the cause of our misunderstandings, we can compensate by explaining why we think differently and by being more patient. For example, we may become more aware of our direct communication style and either explain this fact to people at the outset of each relationship or try to develop a smoother communication style with light social banter.

Some people describe the communication of autistic people as 'spiky', 'prickly' or 'angular', rather than as a smooth, meandering flow of speech. Sometimes treatment of the individual's mental health issues – typically anger, depression, anxiety and stress – leads to relaxation and smoother communication.

Knowing our legal rights

Laws have been drafted in many countries to protect and care for adults who are on the autism spectrum. For example, the Autism Act 2009 was passed in the UK to facilitate the diagnostic pathway for adults and post-diagnostic treatment and care. Also, the National Institute of Health and Care Excellence (www.nice.org.uk) provides guidelines to support health care professionals in the provision of the best possible service to autistic adults in the UK. In the USA, the Combating Autism Act (2006) and Combating Autism Reauthorization Act (2011) authorise ASD research and services throughout the Department of Health and Human Services (HHS).

Autistic adults who are aware of their intellectual disability have access to legal protection by law. On the other hand, it follows that adults who have not identified their intellectual condition would probably not be aware of their legal rights.

Finding suitable employment

The UK Equality Act 2010 and UN Convention protect disabled people from discrimination in the workplace (see www.gov.uk/rights-disabled-person/employment), and a growing number of employers are allocating jobs specifically for disabled people. Adults who know about their intellectual disability should be aware of these 'inclusive' employers, specialist recruitment agencies and governmental support services that facilitate the employment of disabled people.

For example, the international software company SAP decided in 2013 to allocate 1 per cent of their jobs globally to people on the autism spectrum (see http://global.sap.com/corporate-en/news.epx?PressID=20938). Some other employers, for example Specialisterne, employ mainly people who have ASD. Specialisterne, which means 'The Specialists' in Danish, is a social enterprise that provides work for diagnosed adults as business consultants in the field of software testing, programming and data entry for the public and private sectors. The company harnesses the 'gifts', special characteristics and talents of people with autism and secures them meaningful employment, and it has operations in numerous locations around the world (see www.specialisterne.com). A growing number of recruiters match talented disabled people with 'inclusive' employers. For example, Jane Hatton established Evenbreak, a not-for-profit social enterprise, to help disabled jobseekers find work with employers who value their skills (see www.evenbreak.co.uk). Equal Approach (see www.equalapproach.com) is another example of a 'diversity solutions provider'.

Two logos to look out for during our job search are 'Mindful Employer' (with a single tick symbol) and 'Positive about Disabled People' (which contains two tick symbols). Any employer who subscribes to these accreditation systems should treat all employees equally without any discrimination towards disabled people, and should encourage disabled people to apply for jobs at their organisations and help them to realise their full potential.

Getting documentary evidence from a professional as validation

Unfortunately, sometimes it can be challenging to persuade our family and friends that we have this hidden intellectual condition. Many parents of people who have AS do not want to believe that their genes created an autistic being. Many parents do not want to acknowledge any responsibility for their disabled child, so they may resist the truth that the psychiatric condition is primarily inherited genetically.

A medical doctor asked me whether I considered ASD to be an affliction or an advantage. This is a complex question because the answer depends upon whether the autistic adult has access to adequate support and resources. So if we are supported properly, ASD can be an advantage, but without support, ASD may be considered an affliction in neurotypical society. Another point is that most people do not believe what cannot be proven. Many people are sceptical of hidden neurological conditions, even after diagnostic validation by a professional psychiatrist; however, even if others dismiss our diagnosis, the diagnosis surely provides us with peace of mind: *at least we know the truth!* After many years of suffering and bewilderment, we must acknowledge to ourselves that we have finally identified the source of our problems (and gifts, too).

Finding a rational explanation for past issues

Autistic people are logical thinkers, so we often need to understand why things happen the way they do. The diagnosis, and all the information that comes with it, shows us very clearly why we have experienced such bizarre lives. Here are some examples of the insights we may have after receiving our diagnosis:

- People who are on the autism spectrum tend to have impaired theory of mind (or cognitive empathy), so we have difficulty perceiving other people's agendas, thoughts and feelings. This explains why we had so many misunderstandings in the past! Armed with this knowledge, we can be more discerning about with whom we share our life and in whom we confide.

- We may have always sensed that we are 'not good enough' for our parents, without understanding why. The diagnosis finally clears up this issue: our parents could never accept that they gave birth to an autistic child. Now we know the truth!

- When we identify ourselves as intellectual thinkers, we begin to understand why we have big ideas without the ability to materialise them. Many people who have ASD excel in academia because the environment is liberal and there is less demand for multitasking, executive planning, delegation and team playing. Our diagnosis helps us to ground ourselves and consider practical options for living with ASD.

Gaining awareness of the law of attraction

The popular idiom 'birds of a feather flock together' is relevant to people who have ASD. After we understand our neurological condition, we may realise that many of our current or previous friends, acquaintances and even heroes have ASD, too. My diagnosis enabled me to be aware that many of my friends (past and present) are autistic. I was even able to identify the path of autism in my family, so I realised that I was not alone in the family with this condition. My favourite artists, writers, actors and musicians also tended to have ASD.

Understanding ourselves better

Our diagnosis usually provides evidence that we have sound minds, thereby eliminating any fears that we may be insane. Autism spectrum disorder is simply a different way of thinking and behaving which we cannot change. So this realisation should come as a relief.

The diagnosis may bring awareness of the 'social model' of disability, which states that an adverse environment is a major cause of mental ill health among autistic people. Again, this knowledge enables us to forgive ourselves, knowing that any secondary mental disorders (such as anxiety and depression) are caused primarily by external influences.

Enhanced self-knowledge supports self-forgiveness because now we are aware of our challenges and the prejudice that we have always faced in life.

Improving our relationships

Those of us who are in relationships can gain access to lots of self-help guides that can improve the quality of these relationships. When both parties in a relationship are confused and constantly misunderstood, the stress can break up the relationship. Post-diagnostic support provides a roadmap for sustainable living, and this is bound to improve all of our relationships.

The disadvantages of diagnosis

The cost of diagnosis

Many adults in the UK obtain their diagnosis within the NHS because the service is free of charge, although there may be a long waiting period; however, some adults pay for their diagnosis privately and this may cost as much as US$3000, or up to £2000 in the UK. Other than speed, and confidentiality (because the report would not need to be included in our official medical records), there are not really any other benefits of having a private diagnosis.

The risk of misdiagnosis

There is always a risk that the diagnosis, which is essentially a professional opinion, is incorrect, so the opinion may be quashed subsequently. Since the APA changed the diagnostic criteria for ASD (which includes Asperger syndrome) in May 2013, some adults previously diagnosed with Asperger syndrome (ASD) may not fulfil the new criteria for ASD contained in *DSM-5*.

Some people will never be convinced

Even a positive diagnosis by the nation's top psychiatrist will not convince certain types of people about our condition. This is usually the case with parents of autistic people who do not want to consider the reality of their own personalities. It is crucial that we remove any doubt about our personalities because we need to understand our true self. Unfortunately, our condition is potentially hidden, so some conservative or insensitive people are unlikely to believe us.

'Coming out' blunders

After self-identification as a person who has ASD, it's important to be careful about in whom we confide. The widespread ignorance and misunderstanding surrounding autism and ASD cannot be overemphasised. Many people are prejudiced towards autistic people, and the media is partially responsible for the negative public opinion of autistic people as criminals; therefore, if we confide in an untrustworthy person, they may spread malicious gossip that we are insane. So one misguided sharing of confidence may cause the loss of our social life.

Identity-alignment crisis

Self-identification, with or without diagnosis, can lead to a potentially traumatic crisis if we do not have the right post-diagnostic support. Many people are relieved after receiving their positive diagnosis of ASD; however, others have to contend with mental health issues and a drastic loss of self-confidence while struggling to accept a new identity as a disabled person.

> Very late diagnosis of AS can cause a mental breakdown or traumatic crisis. Their whole concept of self and explanation for past experiences – the scaffolding that kept them going – has now gone. It's a huge paradigm shift with an alternative that they have yet to discover and use constructively. There is a mind–body division – a difficulty of the brain connecting to the physical body – and this will be extenuated during this crisis, so the person is likely to be in a very psychologically confused state, needing support and understanding, which is often not available. The diagnostician should explain why the person was bullied and confused in the past, as well as explain how their gifts can help them for the future. However, many clinicians in the UK lack the necessary knowledge. They may know how to perform the diagnosis, but they don't understand the Aspie mind. (Tony Attwood, interview, 24 October 2013)

If the diagnosis causes a traumatic crisis, we may be unable to function normally, which means that we probably will not be fit for work for a while. Financial insecurity usually exacerbates anxiety, stress and depression, especially for autistic people who need more security than neurotypical people. Furthermore, if we identify our personality condition late in life, we may not be hopeful of supporting ourselves during our final years.

Chapter 5 provides some personal insights into how the aforementioned advantages and disadvantages have affected late-diagnosed adults, as they discuss their experiences of both relief and crisis. The chapter also explains an established five-stage psychological model of the process that the newly diagnosed adult may experience as well as providing a shamanic healer's perspective.

Chapter 5

COMMON REACTIONS TO VERY LATE DIAGNOSIS OF AUTISM SPECTRUM DISORDER

People react in many different ways to a late diagnosis of ASD. Some people experience extreme crisis, trauma or even meltdown, whereas many individuals experience relief after receiving a positive diagnosis because, at last, we have identified our true self after many years of soul-searching. *Remember, it is not possible to live an authentic and happy life when we are not aware of our true identity.*

Regardless of our emotional response to this new self-knowledge, our life will never be the same. Our old, bewildered self dies and a new, clearer, real self is born; however, there is bound to be a period of readjustment while we grieve the loss of our old self and get to know our new self. This is a transformational event which Michael John Carley describes as, 'beyond most people's imaginations' (Carley 2008, Introduction).

> My initial feeling after my diagnosis was elation for being vindicated after many years of my family and acquaintances believing that I am like this by choice. After doing some research into ASD I realized that my 'symptoms' or issues matched perfectly...including the way I feel and the things I do, so it seems as though every aspect of my personality, my thoughts and emotions are symptoms of ASD. I felt like I had just discovered that I'm a robot after believing myself to be

human for so many years. My discovery explained everything! I wasn't a prototype but a popular production model. (Anon, www.wrongplanet.net 2013)

Tony Attwood describes the probable consequences of very late diagnosis of Asperger syndrome

Psychopathology, depression, issues of legal and illegal drugs to self-medicate, stress, anxiety disorders, medical disorders due to stress (such as gastrointestinal problems, headaches and exhaustion), issues related to career choices and success, and relationship issues are probable consequences of very late diagnosis of Asperger syndrome. There can also be issues of anger management, because you either internalise it and blame yourself, causing an implosion, or explode with anger towards others for being illogical or inconsistent. The risk for individuals with such high levels of anxiety and being aware of their social confusion is to reduce anxiety and create a bubble of security and safety through use of alcohol and marijuana. Initially these drugs serve as medication for anxiety but also as relaxants in social situations (or to make us 'comfortably numb'). This combination of self-medication can be dangerous for people with AS because in order to cope, they need to use their frontal lobe. The frontal lobe is dissolved (deactivated) by alcohol and marijuana; therefore, the part of the brain that is needed for social reasoning is deactivated after using these substances, so their coping mechanism has been removed.

The value of antidepressants lies in their quality and being less dangerous because intoxication does not occur. They affect different people in different ways so side effects can vary enormously – therefore, it is very important to choose the right type of antidepressant. The person needs help with emotional management. I would prefer that patients use prescribed drugs rather than misuse legal or illegal drugs. I also advocate psychological support for dealing with emotions. (Tony Attwood, interview, 24 October 2013)

The AANE cites relief, anger, denial and accusation as typical responses to the diagnosis. Relief is characterised by the thought *I've always known there was something different about me!*, whereas the thought *Why did no one ever tell me before? I've lost so much time and opportunity from not knowing!* is likely to provoke feelings of anger. Moreover, some recently diagnosed autistic people may defend themselves by accusing other members of their family of having similar personality issues.

Figure 5.1 is adapted from our survey (Wylie and Heath 2013) and shows the types of reactions to late diagnosis that were experienced by adult respondents in the UK.

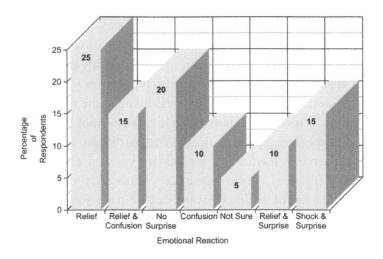

Figure 5.1 Initial reaction to ASD diagnosis

In our survey, the majority of respondents reacted *positively* to their late diagnosis. For instance, 20 per cent of the survey respondents reported no surprise when they received their ASD diagnosis because they had already suspected it; however, one respondent said she was shocked when she received her diagnosis even though she had had her suspicions, while another person commented that 'the light bulb turned on' and he felt happiness and relief when he received his ASD diagnosis. The comments in the next few paragraphs are a sample of those that we received through our survey (Wylie and Heath 2013).

John Carlisle said that he experienced relief, confusion and anger simultaneously after his diagnosis of ASD because he suspected that he would not be able to receive adequate support from the NHS. A major concern for adults who are diagnosed very late in life is money, because the majority of us are underemployed and without any contact with family. Financial insecurity and lack of money exacerbates mental ill health, primarily depression, insomnia and anxiety, so the anxiety caused by social interaction can be compounded by financial worries.

Some autistic adults need a lot of 'downtime' to reflect upon their life and consider their options for the future. For example, Chris Stevens, who experienced relief and confusion after his diagnosis, said he needed some time to get used to his new self-identity, but the diagnosis made sense and he could live with it. Another respondent commented, 'I knew I was different but I did not know why, so I felt relief (after the diagnosis) because I wanted to know the reason why' (Wylie and Heath 2013, p.22).

A key advantage of diagnosis, based on the findings from our survey (Wylie and Heath 2013), is that it helps to explain past issues, such as misunderstandings, broken relationships, bullying, abuse, and failures in the job market; however, some of us may feel that the health system and our family have betrayed us, leaving us with little time left to rebuild a new life. Naturally, such thoughts can lead to anger and resentment, which we should avoid, if possible.

Respondent Carol-Anne said that her diagnosis enabled her to see the world differently:

> Most of my anxiety and depression comes from a feeling that I cannot cope with society; from others feeling that I can be told off, whereas they can't; and that I can be bullied, but not them. Now I recognise my inability to 'be myself' in front of other people because I mimic their behaviour patterns and ways of communicating. This can be detrimental to those closest to me and I don't like myself for doing it. I want to take positive steps to find people who don't make me feel like that, and who make me feel special as I am. (Wylie and Heath 2013, p.22)

Another respondent, Mark Lydon, said, 'All my prayers have been answered; however, I am annoyed with the psychiatrist for not helping me (long ago), but also surprised, because mum is understanding me better now, so she is more relaxed with me now' (Wylie and Heath 2013, p.22).

Another respondent, Fred Smith, said that he felt relief initially, '…although lately I have felt quite confused and bewildered by my situation' (Wylie and Heath 2013, p.22).

A possible reason why the majority of survey respondents reacted to their diagnosis positively is that, according to our survey, 45 per cent of them had been misdiagnosed (and given inappropriate medical treatment) previously; however, whatever the reason, it is generally good to know ourselves better. Yet, at the same time, 80 per cent of our respondents said that they have contemplated suicide, and some engage in self-harm (Wylie and Heath 2013). It's clear that if we are diagnosed late in life, we should be prepared to experience a whole range of emotional responses to this life-changing news.

Autistic adults, particularly older people who may have been in denial about their condition, may experience a traumatic identity crisis, which may involve depression, suicidal thoughts and meltdowns. This crisis may last from a few weeks to months or even years, and in a few cases, some late-diagnosed adults may never fully recover.

Meltdowns

Some adults may be deeply shocked and traumatised by their diagnosis, and they may experience meltdowns. Meltdowns are uncontrollable, involuntary emotional outbursts that occur due to the individual's inability to cope with sensory overload, anger and/or other adverse factors that are present in their personal environment. A tantrum, on the other hand, is a negative emotional outburst that is intended to cause suffering to another person; therefore, tantrums are intentional, manipulative, unreasonable and potentially abusive, whereas meltdowns are involuntary.

Meltdowns are potentially dangerous – particularly when we are alone and without any emotional support – because we may say or do things which we regret later. We may be acutely aware of various forms of abuse that we have experienced inside and outside of our family, and with confirmation of our condition comes the demand 'I want justice *now*!'

During my post-diagnostic crisis, I made several claims for compensation and damages against various parties, including ex-employers. Remember, many autistic individuals have a 'bee in our bonnet' about justice and equity. So, during a meltdown, after excess pressure has built up inside our intellectual bubble, our bubble explodes and we may say or do anything without being in control. It must be quite scary for others to witness a meltdown.

Is it fair to judge an autistic person's behaviour if he or she is experiencing a mental breakdown or meltdown?

Neurotypical people have never experienced ASD, so their attitude is 'Pull yourself together!' or 'Calm down!' without realising that it's not going to work. For many years the individual with ASD has experienced intense emotions, and when they receive the diagnosis there is a paradigm shift and a complete re-evaluation of self. The trauma of this paradigm shift affects people in different ways. Some people are relieved, whereas others are traumatised if they feel uncertain about the future, because most people with ASD find it difficult to adjust to change; however, there can be a sense of euphoria after realising that you are not psychotic or mad. In any case, positive diagnosis brings all the emotions to the fore of 'Why do I have to deal with this so late in my life? This should have been identified by professionals in the past. How will my life change because now I have to explain myself to people who don't seem to understand my problems?' People with ASD are not good at describing their inner thoughts and feelings to others. Often this means that emotions are swirling around in the person's mind but are difficult to grasp, define and disclose to others. So the person is going through all sorts of changes and they need lots of support. After diagnosis, the person needs counselling to come to terms with his or her revised self-image, but often diagnosticians don't offer such services. (Tony Attwood, interview, 24 October 2013)

Older people who have been diagnosed very late in their lives are most vulnerable to meltdowns, particularly those who are trying to cling onto their previous self-image of normality. Also, older people are more likely to have internalised unfair beliefs about disabled people, meaning that we can literally become victims of our own prejudice; however, it is possible to remove these disempowering beliefs, possibly with the support of a psychotherapist or shamanic healer.

On a positive note, if you ever experience a meltdown, you will probably discover who your genuine friends are. Also, try to remember that meltdowns are part of the transformational process – stepping stones towards self-acceptance of our new self – so we should not necessarily judge them as 'bad'. Let's forgive ourselves for our meltdowns!

Confusion

It is normal for recently diagnosed adults to experience confusion and bewilderment, because initially we lack knowledge about ASD. As mentioned earlier, there is a massive amount of misinformation about autism out there, so many aspects of our new self-identity may be confusing.

The way out of the confusion is to communicate and ask for support from genuinely knowledgeable autism practitioners and to access reliable sources of information about ASD. The best practitioners to consult are those who work as full-time autism specialists. It is also very helpful to attend a regular ASD support group and to get support from an ASD mentor.

Do read as many of the relevant books as possible published by Jessica Kingsley Publishers, who specialise in books about the autism spectrum. Also recommended are established experts, such as Simon Baron-Cohen, Luke Beardon, Tony Attwood and Michael Fitzgerald. Some of the most cutting-edge wisdom is emerging from Sheffield Hallam University. Also, consult the websites of the main national autism organisations, which are listed in the directory at the back of this book.

The way out of confusion is extensive research into ASD using reliable information sources and specialists. Be aware that misinformation can exacerbate confusion and impede recovery, so be discerning always.

Anger

There are many reasons why we may feel angry after discovering our true identity. Whatever our reasons are, it is essential that we do our best to overcome self-destructive emotions as soon as possible. We cannot change our past, but we can influence our future by adopting a positive outlook.

> First, we must forgive ourselves for taking so long to identify our hidden intellectual disability. Ultimately, we should take responsibility for our own lives instead of blaming others for our misguidance. Remember, information about ASD became available in the English language only in 1991, which explains why there is still so much ignorance about it.
>
> Aspies definitely have trouble with emotional regulation. But what is not clearly understood is that some days are better than others. For example, a teacher might say that an autistic child was capable yesterday, and so he is quite capable of doing it today. Wrong! Each day has its different challenges which affect our moods and ability to cope. (Roderick Wintour, correspondence, 10 December 2013)

Autistic people are usually unable to regulate their emotions. Part of the problem is that we tend to focus more on our impairments than our strengths, which is understandable because there is much more information available across the media about our negative traits. Counselling and psychotherapy can help us to balance our perception of our strengths and weaknesses.

Here are just some of the reasons why we may feel intense anger:

- We may think that we have discovered our condition too late in life to do anything about it.

- It's possible that some close friends and family members withheld the truth from us, thus 'robbing' us of opportunities to get our life on track sooner.

- Only now do we understand why we were bullied inside and outside of our families.

- We are indignant at the thought, *Why should I be included in the 1 per cent of the population that is treated as inferior?*

- We have been put through unnecessary confusion and upset due to a series of misdiagnoses.

- We have been living with the frustration of being constantly misunderstood by everyone.

- As adults we are neglected because all the support is directed towards children.

- We don't have enough money or support to rebuild our lives.

Remember, however, that in spite of all the aforementioned difficulties, it's better to reach our goals late rather than never. Many autistic adults go to their grave without understanding themselves. When we understand ourselves and the reasons for our suffering (and after going through the identity-alignment process) we are in a position to eliminate our anger through forgiveness.

Relief

Many late-diagnosed autistic adults react to the ASD diagnosis with relief, because finally, perhaps after receiving several misdiagnoses and inappropriate treatments, we receive a diagnosis that fits our condition and explains our history of relationship problems.

In our UK autism survey, 40 per cent of respondents claimed that they reacted to their ASD diagnosis with relief (Wylie and Heath 2013, p.21). Included in this statistic are 'relief and confusion' (15 per cent) and 'relief and surprise' (10 per cent) (see Figure 5.1).

Jen Birch was both shocked and relieved when she identified ASD in herself:

> I was shocked at the moment of realisation – the eureka moment when I discovered that the list of ASD traits fit me – although it was a positive, happy kind of shock. I also felt intense relief at having found 'the answer' to my life's bewilderment. (Jen Birch, correspondence, 26 November 2012)

Sara Hendrickx describes the typical reactions of her clients to their ASD diagnosis:

> Perhaps 95 per cent of the people that I see following some sort of assessment are incredibly relieved if they wanted the diagnosis. It's a massively positive thing for them. It's a weight lifted off their shoulders. It's amazing. But I always warn people when they get a positive diagnosis to be prepared for a bit of an emotional rollercoaster in the months that follow. Even if you were absolutely delighted about this diagnosis, there will likely be days when you don't believe it's true and you become very angry about things that happened in the past and that nobody noticed you were struggling. Why didn't they notice? You reflect on your life and think about relationships, jobs and things that have failed. This can provoke an enormous amount of sadness and anger. It's a big rollercoaster ride. I always say to people, 'Just sit with this for a while and don't use it in lots of weird and illogical ways.' You get the relief, but with that comes regret, reflection, insecurity and sadness. When I think about things that may or may not have been, and decisions I made which weren't great, it's a bit sad. (Sarah Hendrickx, interview, 20 November 2013)

Mental ill health

Mental ill health is common in adults with ASD who are diagnosed late in life because we have been struggling to survive using intellect instead of intuition and instinct in a neurotypical environment.

You may recall from Chapter 2 that 100 per cent of the respondents to our survey stated that they suffer from anxiety. In addition to the pervasive mental health issues of anxiety, stress, depression and insomnia identified in our survey (see Figure 2.1), 70 per cent of respondents mentioned that they have anger management issues (Wylie and Heath 2013, p.26).

> Mental ill health can be prevented by appropriate and timely intervention during childhood. There would be less chance of developing clinical depression, being bullied, or alcohol and drug use. One of my great concerns is that the psychiatric services for adults really do not understand Asperger syndrome. They need the training as well as the attitude shift, and it is rare for a person with AS to actually benefit from admission to a psychiatric unit. I have never actually encountered a single autistic person who benefited from admission to a psychiatric hospital – and I have been working in this field since the 1970s! Psychiatric units have an adverse affect on people who have AS because the staff don't know about AS and may not understand that Aspies don't work well in groups. Furthermore, the person is in the company of other people who are emotionally challenging, volatile and extreme, which is very upsetting for the person with AS. A psychiatric ward is not relaxing. If you are in one, it's full of people with intense emotions and interpersonal difficulties, and the person with AS does not know intuitively the ground rules of this new culture. So they feel like they are on another planet. I do everything I can to keep people with AS *out* of psychiatric hospitals. (Tony Attwood, interview, 24 October 2013)

It is often agreed that mental ill health may be a costly consequence of not having been diagnosed during childhood or not having received appropriate and timely support. Due to our ability to mentally catalogue past hurts and traumas, when we are bullied or abused, or when we encounter relationship or employment issues, our mental health (including self-esteem) is inevitably affected adversely.

Any person who experiences clinical depression needs treatment for mental health. Sadness, however, is something that people suffer on their own without warranting psychotherapy or medication. One of the clinical hunches I have is the high level of addiction among people with Asperger syndrome (ASD). Alcohol, prescription drugs and illegal drugs are the main substances to which adults become addicted. Pink Floyd refers to this state as 'comfortably numb' in their song of the same title, which is about self-medicating to avoid feeling certain emotions. Alcohol starts off as a mild relaxant, but actually it is a depressant. Some adults who have ASD obtain drugs, such as Valium, and misuse them. Then they may become curious about other drugs, from morphine to heroin, but these people may not be viewed as having AS; instead, they would probably be involved with psychiatric support because their primary concern may be addiction. (Tony Attwood, interview, 13 November 2013)

Other reactions

There are several other ways in which we may react after our late diagnosis. Some undiagnosed adults are known to change their names or adopt various aliases while desperately trying to fathom the truth, and this is often mistaken for schizophrenia or multiple personality disorder. Of course, not understanding our true self can offer unlimited freedom to be whoever we want to be, but adopting more than one personality can be confusing for all parties involved.

Changing names for people with ASD

When I asked Michael Fitzgerald whether it is common for people with ASD to adopt aliases and to have multiple careers, he said that it is, and the cause is identity diffusion. For decades I sensed that I was living in two separate worlds: the realm of 'being', integrity and passion; and the neurotypical world of 'doing', obligation and suffering. I changed my name twice to emphasise new chapters in my life. In 2001, before I left the UK, I used the name Normand; and later, in 2004, I used the name Kristar to support my esoteric interests, including numerology. I also used different pen names. I use different names to aid personal development, not to support any nefarious activities. Changing names can be extremely empowering when exercised with positive intention.

Other people may withdraw from society and many experience a loss of self-esteem, particularly during the crisis period while trying to come to terms with an alternative reality. Autistic people who are particularly vulnerable to low self-esteem are those of us who pretended to be normal and tried hard to fit into society.

Many Aspies adopt aliases but not for the reasons that many people think. It is assumed that people with ASD use aliases to conceal their identity and this is part of the perception that we are antisocial; therefore, we hide behind a false identity. For many of us this is quite incorrect.

I have an alias named Gyro (gyro812 on the Internet). Gyro is a popular name on the Web and there are several people who use the alias gyro812. Gyro was a name given to me by my fellow fire fighters out of respect. I had a reputation as an inventor who thought outside the square, which saved the day and even lives on several occasions. The number 812 was that of the fire engine I used to drive. The name Gyro was always respected and was never used in a derogatory way. As for my real name, I was teased from the beginning of year one back in my school days. Gyro is a name which for me is a symbol of achievement and respect. I have been insulted many times over my real name, which is why I use the alias Gyro.

An Aspie lady I know goes by the alias Princess for similar reasons, and with others it may be related to someone or some character they respect. Sometimes we even mimic the behaviour of others we respect and may call ourselves an alias based on that person; however, I am not aware of anybody (and I know a lot of Aspies!) who uses aliases to conceal who they are on an antisocial level. (Roderick Wintour, correspondence, 10 December 2013)

As discussed earlier, self-harm and suicidal feelings are common responses to late diagnosis, especially when there is no financial or emotional support available. Adults with ASD perceive suicide as a logical solution to a hopeless situation.

> I have a theory about suicide which I have discussed with a number of other Asperger people and they have agreed that it applies to them, too. This is not to trivialise it or suggest that neurotypical people do not experience the same suicidal thoughts as people with AS, who sadly do sometimes determine that acting upon those thoughts is the best or only option open to them at that time. My Aspie opinion of suicidal thinking is maybe just a non-emotional, logical analysis of the situation: suicide is genuinely one of the potential options. I think that neurotypical people can find suicidal thinking very shocking (those who have never considered it), whereas for some of us it's almost a part of everyday life. I think that is probably very hard to get your head around if it's not something with which you are familiar. For me, it's just how it is and has been for as long as I can remember. (Sarah Hendrickx, interview, 20 November 2013)

Be discerning of who you communicate with – especially during identity alignment – because contact with insensitive, ignorant or patronising people can cause us more harm than good. Ideally we should relate with or consult only people who are empathetic and who don't doubt our diagnosis. Some late-diagnosed adults enjoy improved relationships with parents and other relatives following self-identification *if* those relatives are empathetic and willing to face the facts. Those autistic adults who are in relationships with patient, caring and sensitive partners have a massive advantage over single people; however, it is preferable to be single and alone than in an inappropriate relationship. Also, be discerning about which friends you disclose your ASD condition to, because confiding in the wrong person can result in social isolation. (The 'coming out' process is discussed in Chapter 6.)

The milestone of diagnosis represents the beginning of a new self-identity. As shown by the first-hand accounts in this chapter, people react to the realisation of a new identity in different ways; some are relieved, whereas others may be traumatised. Any person who experiences a crisis needs support in various forms: emotional support, counselling, mentoring, coaching and financial support. If these supports are not available during the period of crisis, the risk of suicide or self-harm is much higher, the crisis may be prolonged and there is a higher chance of experiencing mental ill health. To reduce such risks, let us now briefly consider how to create an ideal environment for this transformational experience, a topic which is covered in more detail in Chapter 7.

Mitigating adverse reactions

The recently diagnosed adult needs as much rest and relaxation as possible, ideally with access to genuine friends and supportive family. Many older autistic adults have no parents and may not have any understanding friends or relatives; however, there are numerous local autism support groups in many countries whose members can help us to understand ourselves better and give us the opportunity to build friendships with like-minded people.

During an identity-alignment crisis or mental breakdown, most employed autistic adults would benefit by taking time off work. Expecting a traumatised person to continue working in a stressful job is similar to expecting an aeroplane to reach its next destination on time after it has crashed. Downtime is essential for reflection and to consider how to start a new life.

After diagnosis, mental health issues can cause considerable suffering. A local mental health team may be able to provide specialist support, and they may even provide a part- or full-time support worker. Also, wherever you live, you should be able to benefit from an online mentor or chat with other autistic people on relevant forums (e.g. www.wrongplanet.net).

People who experience an identity crisis should focus on whatever makes them feel happy. It helps to stay in a naturally beautiful and calm place. Do whatever it takes to enhance your emotional well-being. Go wherever there is light!

The crisis begins with the knowledge that we are different and awareness of our ASD condition, and it ends when we have accepted, and feel comfortable with, our new self-identity. Between the start and end of this process, for many if not most of us, there will be some tough days – depression, desperation, sleepless nights and suicidal thinking – but remember to follow the light until the end of the tunnel. Our journey of self-understanding can be explained by some psychological models that track the path of transformation during the identity crisis.

The Kübler-Ross model

Elisabeth Kübler-Ross constructed a five-stage psychological model to explain people's reaction to change in the context of coming to terms with death and dying (Kübler-Ross 2005). Although the Kübler-Ross model focuses on the stages of grief following the death of a loved one, it can also apply to anyone who experiences inner change or identity crisis.

Change inevitably involves some form of loss before we gain something new. When we become aware of our new identity, our original identity (or self-image) dies, so there will be a period of grieving. Afterwards, we begin to construct a new identity that embraces the fact that we are on the autism spectrum.

The five stages in the Kübler-Ross model are denial, anger, bargaining, depression and acceptance. Elisabeth Kübler-Ross believes that these five stages apply to anyone who receives shocking or traumatic news, because these reactions are defence mechanisms or coping strategies. Many older autistic adults react to their self-diagnosis with shock, surprise and even trauma – particularly those of us who believed that we were normal, albeit slightly eccentric, for several decades. The stages in the model and their impact are discussed below.

Denial (stage 1)

The first stage is shock and denial. The information is too painful to accept, so we distance ourselves from it, like an ostrich burying its head in the sand. In our survey, 25 per cent of respondents admitted to being in denial of their condition. One of the respondents said, 'The feelings of maladjustment are so prevalent in late diagnosis that, in a way, you are too scared to believe it' (Wylie and Heath 2013, p.20). So the first stage in the Kübler-Ross model is resistance to accepting the truth of our condition.

Anger (stage 2)

The second stage is anger. It is common, therefore, to feel anger towards many people; for instance, towards parents and employers for bullying, or simply to feel anger that you have ASD. Jen Birch admitted to feeling angry for a short period. She said:

> Creeping in a little later was a feeling of anger that I had reached the age of forty-three [to understand my condition], and I had to experience psychological and other abuse before accidentally finding out what the real issue was. (Jen Birch, interview, 16 November 2012)

Bargaining (stage 3)

Bargaining is another method of avoidance, and it works like this: if I promise to do something specific, can I avoid the change happening to me? The late-diagnosed individual with ASD may resist the paradigm shift towards perceiving oneself as an autistic person by making a bargain such as the following: *If I end my life now, can I avoid the change that is happening?* Apart from bargaining with suicide, drugs or religion, how else can we avoid the transformation in our life?

Depression (stage 4)

Depression is a normal reaction to loss of the old self-identity and worry about how the change will affect the future. 'There are going to be times of depression after receiving a positive diagnosis of ASD, but the overwhelming effect of the self-realisation process should be positive,' says Michael John Carley (interview, 16 November 2012). After his own diagnosis, Michael realised that it was the wiring in his brain that caused his quirky behaviour, not his character. Instead of carrying on pretending to be neurotypical, this valuable self-knowledge enabled him to access various resources (both online and offline) to validate his condition. As Michael says, 'Maintaining pretence of normality can often be disempowering.'

After Michael's formal diagnosis, his anticipated relief at having such a weight lifted from his shoulders suddenly disappeared. He remembers standing on the sidewalk experiencing a barrage of negative thoughts and describes this moment of sadness in his book:

> In that moment of diagnosis, the euphoria I'd predicted and started to feel was quickly metamorphosing into a fast-moving hurricane of negativity – a monumental sadness with the realization that, 'Yes, you were all alone your whole life! You do not belong in the same category as these other people! You do not have that sense of shared experience…with anyone!' (Carley 2008)

However, Michael, who has always had a strong sense of self-worth, did not remain in that dark place for long. His experience was much smoother than most. Typically, post-diagnostic depression lasts between 2 and 6 months.

Acceptance (stage 5)

Acceptance marks the end of the identity crisis, when the autistic person finally accepts himself or herself. Part of the process requires the individual to remove any internalised negative beliefs, to be mindful of the positive 'gifts' available to us and to forgive ourselves for resisting the truth of our identity for so long. Of course, we also probably have numerous people and organisations to forgive for the mistreatment we received over several decades.

The four stages of response to a new self-identity

An alternative four-stage model, which is an adaptation of the Kübler-Ross model, is as follows:

1. Shock and denial – when we immediately reject the idea of a different self-image.

2. Anger and depression – common responses to change and instability that we cannot control, which can cause feelings of powerlessness and despair.

3. Exploration and insight – when we can see all the options available to us (i.e. 'the big picture') after realising that change is inevitable, and can identify an appropriate way forward with a new self-identity.

4. Resolution to accept the change and our new circumstances – after experiencing stages 1–3, we can embrace our new self and take positive steps to improve our lives.

Luke Beardon says that most of his clients feel different initially and usually experience depression after their diagnosis, until they finally accept themselves:

> Obviously, each person reacts in their own unique way, but there are some patterns. Very often, the individual is extremely relieved *if* the process is one of positivity rather than negativity. I think that it depends on how the diagnostic process is handled; if performed well, with respect for the individual and promotion of the benefits of ASD, the individual can feel hugely empowered. For example, rather than use the term 'diagnosis', it is much better to use the word 'identity'. The connotations of the two terms are very different conceptually, and such issues can have a major (positive or negative) impact on the individual. The person may also feel a huge sense of relief

– a 'so that explains everything' type of sentiment. As noted, though, this depends on the process and the post-diagnostic support on offer.

Many people feel very low at some point after their diagnosis, such as bitterness over why their condition wasn't identified earlier. Another common reason for feeling depressed involves wondering whether an earlier diagnosis could have made a difference. Most people go through a process of recalling significant life events and almost reliving them, but from a different perspective. Some people experience a grieving process as they realise that they are not who they thought they were. (Luke Beardon, personal communication, 31 January 2013)

A shamanic healer's perspective

Altazar Rossiter, a shamanic healer, has helped many clients to accept their authentic identity during periods of change and crisis. According to Altazar, we construct a rigid self-identity at an early age, and then formulate core beliefs to reinforce our belief in our self-image. When we have to change our self-identity, the experience of trauma and confusion is inevitable, as he explains:

> We construct our identity mostly during pre-linguistic sensory (feeling) experiences. We try to interpret these experiences to make sense of our relationship with the external world. There is nothing absolute about this, and we don't need linguistic or reasoning abilities to make revisions to our self-identity, so our behavioural patterns tend to be entrenched and difficult to reach with a rational linguistic approach.
>
> Our self-identity goes hand in glove with the core beliefs that we develop about ourselves and the way the world is. Subsequently, we view the world through the interpretive lens of the identity we create, and that recreates and reinforces our belief structures. We have already anchored (our core beliefs) in the story we have told ourselves, so we map that story onto what we perceive as our existence. I would see the diagnosis of any – what might be called

abnormal – condition as presenting a serious challenge to the identity you might have created. This could be very traumatic. It would necessarily involve a complete revision of everything you knew about yourself and how you fit (or don't fit) into the world; however, there is a potential opportunity to deconstruct the old false identity and move into a deeper truth of being. This would be nothing less than transformational. Once any residual resentments or shame have been let go, it could provide a wonderful doorway to a more fulfilling life.

Be careful about labels. For instance, I would encourage you to say that you have 'a form of Asperger syndrome (ASD)' rather than 'I am an ASD sufferer' or 'a bit autistic'. The [ASD] condition is something you live with rather than what you are. Avoid any 'I am' statement that carries the suggestion that you are broken in any way.

Your existential paradigm – how you define yourself within the context of the reality you perceive around you – has shifted for good. And I reckon *good* is the right word. (Altazar Rossiter, correspondence, 29 November 2012)

Chapter 6

THE 'COMING OUT'
PROCESS

The 'coming out' process is part of the healing process, which occurs during, or even after, our identity-alignment process. Remember that identity alignment begins with the tipping point – when self-identification is irreversible – and ends when we accept our new identity.

There are several variables inherent in the coming-out process: timing, manner of communication and the person(s) in whom we confide. There is no right or wrong way of coming out, although each choice carries its own risk. Most individuals who have Asperger syndrome are likely to come out in one of the following ways:

- during a meltdown, after the 'tipping point' of self-identification

- during the exploration and information-gathering stage, prior to diagnosis

- after a positive diagnosis or pre-diagnostic assessment

- after we have chosen a suitable lifestyle or plan for the remainder of our life

- when we have completely accepted our condition and revised self-image.

Of these manifestations, probably the most inappropriate time to come out is during a meltdown, shortly after self-identification, because a meltdown is usually driven by anger and confusion, so we may regret some of the things that we say later. A safer time to come out is after we have effectively researched our new identity, when we feel comfortable with our condition.

Be aware that, even with a formal diagnosis from the most respected psychiatrist, there will still be people who doubt your claim. As Michael John Carley says, many parents and relatives may not feel comfortable discussing the origin of our neurological condition (interview, 16 November 2012).

Misinformation on the Internet

When I confided in one of my friends about my newly identified condition, I received the following response:

'This is just a lot of [impolite word] bull. Believe it or not, I have never heard about anybody who suddenly *got* Asperger syndrome (ASD) – it's a mental disease you are either born with or not. I had to use Google [a lot] to find this out.' This response reveals two major avenues of misinformation. First, most people do not realise that there are millions of undiagnosed autistic adults who have lived with ASD all their lives. An undiagnosed adult with ASD may become aware of their condition during their lifetime, but many go to their grave without this knowledge.

Second, the response shows that my friend believes that Asperger syndrome (ASD) is a mental disease, which confirms that the Internet is rife with false information. As mentioned earlier, mental illness is a secondary psychiatric condition caused by adverse environmental issues and lack of appropriate support.

My neurotypical 'friend' who searched the Web for (mis) information about ASD has above-average intelligence and two tertiary degrees, so he is neither stupid nor uneducated. I wonder what less intelligent and less educated people would make of ASD after a 30-minute Internet session!

Of course, the safest and possibly most sensible time to come out is when we have completely accepted our new self-image;

however, this is 'easier said than done' because the crisis period usually involves many intense and painful feelings. Also, one of the prominent characteristics of ASD is saying whatever is on our mind without any effective filter to protect us (and others). This means that it is difficult for us to keep secrets, and once we realise our real identity, it would seem like a massive breach of integrity to hide our inner truth.

The method of communication we use when we come out also influences the responses we receive. The main advice is to communicate as clearly, logically and smoothly as possible. One major pitfall to avoid is communicating such emotive issues while under the influence of anger or alcohol (or any other mood-altering substance). Also, remember that conflict is often easier to deal with via email rather than by telephone or face to face.

The key groups of people that we might want to 'come out' with are:

- parents and relatives (if they are still alive)
- potential employers
- friends and acquaintances
- current or potential relationship partners.

Figure 6.1 is from our survey (Wylie and Heath 2013, p.23) and shows who our respondents told about their late diagnosis.

Our survey revealed that approximately 66 per cent of the respondents told their parents, relatives, friends, employers and potential relationship partners about their ASD condition (Wylie and Heath 2013, p.23). But bear in mind that many of us are in contact with very few people.

A possible explanation for the high prevalence of coming out to all parties is that many adults with ASD only have contact with other autistic individuals, perhaps at a local support group. The respondents' friends who have ASD would not use the information against them, as some neurotypical people might do, even inadvertently.

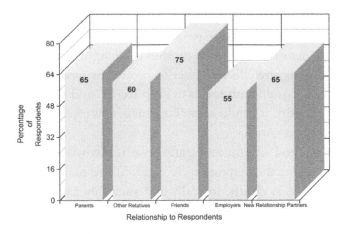

Figure 6.1 Coming out as having ASD

Key groups of people in whom we might choose to confide

Parents and relatives

Older autistic adults do not usually receive an empathetic response from parents and relatives because of their ingrained beliefs, 'stiff upper lip' and inflexibility. Most parents and relatives of late-diagnosed adults do not want to be associated with any form of autism, even though they may know that ASD is primarily inherited genetically. Unfortunately, the medical model for autism (which is consistent with behavioural therapy) encourages people to deny their condition and pretend to be neurotypical.

The medical model for autism is based upon the premise that if an autistic person acts like a neurotypical person, they have been cured; however, this model does not take account of the resulting damage to the individual's mental health and self-esteem. The medical model may work for successful autistic adults who have a sound support network with adequate resources.

In ideal circumstances, every disabled child has parents who are able to explain to them about their developmental disability and provide the necessary support; however, if adults with ASD have been left to discover their differences on their own, in most cases their parents are probably too old, conservative and inflexible in their thinking to accept the truth when it is revealed. In such cases, coming out with parents is humiliating and frustrating, causing further estrangement.

Jen Birch's disclosure to her mother

Jen Birch waited an entire year before she told her mum about her diagnosis because she didn't want to upset her. Jen states:

> As it happened, it did not upset her, but only confirmed her feeling – which had started as soon as I was born – she told me that something was different about me. Mum has been extremely supportive towards me; all the more since hearing my diagnosis. (Birch 2003, p.243)

Jen admits that she feels lucky that her mum reacted in such a positive way.

A vitally important aspect of the healing process is the information collected about the psychiatric disorders in the family. A thorough investigation of the psychological profiles of all first-, second- and third-degree family members should be mandatory. It is essential that we understand how we inherited our condition to explain the communication problems within our family. My mother commented on many occasions about the constant fighting between her husband and his father, and between her husband and son. Only after my late diagnosis and considerable research into the family did I begin to understand the reasons for these problematic relationships.

One way of identifying psychiatric conditions is to observe each person's best friends and personal heroes, because like minds attract one another. For example, narcissistic people tend to respect fellow narcissists. Likewise, people who have ASD are typically attracted to those who have autism. However, neurodiversity is complex, and in some cases, there can be an overlap between ASD and Narcissistic Personality Disorder (NPD).

If you are a late-diagnosed individual and your parents are alive, it can be very helpful to identify the genetic path of autism in your family, and therefore it is necessary to ask some awkward questions.

Employers

In general, our chances of getting an employment contract are much slimmer if we express ourselves transparently. Sadly, due to the prevailing ignorance about ASD across society, it still pays to tell white lies about our neurotype. Tony Attwood says, 'Men with Asperger syndrome can also be admired for speaking their minds, having a sense of social justice and strong moral convictions' (Attwood 2006, Chapter 13). So it is much more difficult for people who are on the autism spectrum to tell lies, even white lies. Inevitably, we 'shoot ourselves in the foot' by being overly transparent and consequently lose potential opportunities.

Unfortunately, the negative stigma attached to the autism label is everywhere. Rod Morris, who has ASD and is studying for an MA in Autism at Sheffield Hallam University, states:

> There is a stigma. I have educated many local authorities and organisations and have found that people have difficulty seeing someone with autism as being a professional. The majority of autism charities just want to use people like me for free information, while the remunerative contracts are reserved for neurotypical professionals. (Rod Morris, interview, 27 February 2013)

Another matter of concern is that in many social enterprises, charities and autism support organisations, autistic people are under-represented among their staff. Surely, autism charities would benefit by employing people who have first-hand experience of ASD. Employers benefit massively by treating autistic people as healthy human beings and adjusting the work environment to enable us to be fully productive.

Employers that promote themselves as equal opportunity, mindful or inclusive employers are not necessarily to be trusted as such because these organisational 'badges' are essentially purchased through an accreditation process so that they can portray themselves positively to customers and other stakeholders. (In a similar vein, many companies have pretended to be environmentally friendly to gain favour with environmentally friendly customers.) Remember that the actual decision makers in the recruitment process may not be quite as empathetic towards autistic people as their corporate employer portrays itself to be.

Regardless of whether you tell your potential employer about your ASD condition, it is beneficial to explain to recruiters your key strengths. Typical positive traits of autistic people are the ability to focus on a single task for a long time, above-average intelligence, adept systemisation skills, goal orientation, ability to see 'the wood for the trees', abstract thinking ability and integrity.

Autism expert Dennis Debbaudt recommends 'soft disclosure', which may be considered as the middle way (2002). Soft disclosure is the communication of our key strengths and weaknesses without mentioning specific diagnostic labels (such as ASD). This method of coming out is practical because the individual who discloses his or her condition softly is being transparent and ethical but not scaring people by using psychiatric labels that most people associate with madness. If you decide to tell your potential employer about your ASD condition, it may be a good idea to wait until the final stage of the recruitment process. Coming out at the outset of the job application process would probably limit our chances of being invited for an interview, unless the employer is specifically looking for an autistic employee.

Sometimes being honest about our neurological condition with employers can be beneficial, particularly if they support accommodations at work for people who have disabilities. An increasing number of employers, particularly computer software companies, are actively seeking autistic employees who are hard-working and focused.

Jen Birch says she told potential employers about her ASD condition at the interview stage, and eventually she was offered a suitable job. Of course, Jen's approach increases the risk of rejection, but naturally she felt better about herself by being open and truthful about her condition (Birch 2003).

Try to perceive the situation from the employer's viewpoint. Employers want hard-working, reliable, productive employees who add value to their shareholders' investment. We know that autistic people can be hard-working, productive and focused. Most of us are goal-oriented, honest (to a fault) and good at keeping appointments and meeting deadlines; however, we are sometimes difficult to work with because we misunderstand people (and vice versa), and we usually need to work in our own unique way. We may be direct in our communications and impatient to 'get to the point'. Also, our quirky or 'freaky' ways intimidate some people.

Friends and acquaintances

It probably pays to be discerning about the friends and acquaintances we 'come out' to because many people are influenced by the negative press about people who are autistic. Many people only want to associate with other healthy and successful people, which is understandable as a survival strategy. Remember, there is a massive amount of misinformation about Asperger syndrome, and most people confuse ASD with mental illness, and few people want to have friends who are mentally ill. Even doctors and psychiatrists believe that ASD is a disorder or disease, so what chance does the lay public have of understanding this potentially hidden condition?

Some friends and acquaintances would disbelieve us anyway if we told them about our condition. It's understandable because ASD is a hidden intellectual disability and some of us may appear to be completely normal, albeit slightly eccentric. Our friends may incorrectly assume that such psychiatric conditions are always identified during childhood. Therefore, it may be a challenge to explain why we have been unaware of our condition for several decades; an excellent article to show these sceptics is that by Simon Baron-Cohen and colleagues (Baron-Cohen *et al.* 2007).

We must also remember that gossip and inaccurate rumours can ruin a person's social life, so it is important to consider the consequences of telling any friend. As mentioned earlier, a single 'coming out' blunder can cost us our entire social life.

If possible, it is best to come out to friends and acquaintances on a highly discerning basis, and preferably *after* we have accepted our condition fully; however, this advice is not necessarily easy to apply, especially during meltdowns or crises, when it's nigh on impossible to control ourselves.

Also, many autistic people have enough trouble knowing who our true friends are anyway, due to lack of cognitive empathy, so we can easily confide in the wrong people (those who misunderstand ASD). Moreover, as mentioned previously, we find it difficult to keep secrets, preferring to be open and fully transparent about who we are. Several respondents in our survey said they would tell everyone about their condition because they are not ashamed of it. For example, John Carlisle says, 'I've nothing to hide; I am what I am' (Wylie and Heath 2013, p.23).

Overall, it's the individual's choice, but if we share our revelations with friends, we must ensure that they are properly informed about ASD; therefore, if possible, we should wait to tell selected friends after we understand ourselves better and are in a position to explain our situation to them clearly.

Current or potential relationship partners

The majority of autistic adults who are diagnosed late in life tend to live alone without a relationship partner or carer; however, many autistic adults identify their condition via their relationship partner. If you are in a relationship, make sure you and your partner read *Alone Together: Making an Asperger Marriage Work* by Katrin Bentley (2007). This book explains the challenges faced by both the person with ASD and the neurotypical person in a 'mixed' relationship. Of course, it is necessary to discuss any psychiatric issues with a current partner at the earliest possible opportunity; otherwise, misunderstandings and issues will grow and get out of control.

In the case of a potential relationship partner, it's an individual's decision about when to disclose their ASD condition, although the majority of older autistic men may well have given up on romantic relationships by the time they figure themselves out. Remember, also, that there is a tendency for people who have neurological conditions, such as ASD, to attract others with similar conditions. For example, I attracted relationship partners who had bipolar disorder, narcissistic personality disorder and attachment disorder, as well as ASD. On a positive note, such couples should have lots to talk about, assuming both parties are willing to 'come out'. If either partner wants to have children, obviously it's very important to discuss the potential genetic issues. It is noteworthy that autistic children can be happy if they are properly cared for, and some of the happiest adults with ASD have children.

Conclusion

How we come out, and with whom, is the individual's choice, so there is no single clear-cut solution. At one end of the coming-out spectrum is Jen Birch, who says, 'For me, it is a case of that saying of Jesus: "The truth will set you free". Getting rid of that one big secret certainly makes me feel liberated' (Birch 2003); however, Liane Holliday Willey's mother holds the view that: 'The truth may set you free, but it doesn't necessarily set everyone else free' (Murray 2006). At the other end of the coming-out spectrum are autistic people in senior positions – typically doctors, researchers, lecturers, scientists and engineers – who choose to tell nobody for fear of being a victim of the prevailing stigmas and possibly losing their career status.

After experiencing some of the feelings (not all negative) and consequences as a result of receiving a late diagnosis, how can we live with our condition and look to a brighter future? Chapter 7 explores some tried and tested coping strategies that can open the door to a more fulfilling future.

Chapter 7

HOW TO LIVE WELL WITH VERY LATE DIAGNOSIS OF AUTISM SPECTRUM DISORDER

This final chapter provides practical methods and guidance for individuals on the spectrum for leading a good life. This includes access to appropriate support, learning to relax, and building a community of trustworthy friends and carers.

Coping techniques

Probably the most important coping strategy is about understanding our real needs, and then asking appropriate people how we can satisfy them. Historically, it has been considered feminine to express our emotions or to discuss our vulnerabilities. Autistic adults, and particularly men, are especially affected by such damaging cultural programming. Women are arguably better equipped to survive in the modern world due to their enhanced intuition, instinct to survive, and ability to multitask and ask for what they need, whereas men prefer to portray themselves as strong, so they usually find it difficult to admit their vulnerabilities and ask for help. Many autistic adults have been punished many times for asking for what we need, but if we don't reach out and ask for something, we won't get it!

Self-knowledge is everything. Without understanding our mental condition, we are lost and bewildered, without a clue as to why we have so many challenges. Although late diagnosis of ASD can be traumatic, without this vital information about ourselves we are powerless, hopeless and utterly confused. Diagnosis of ASD brings a massive amount of knowledge that serves as a blueprint and enables us to clarify our strengths and weaknesses, opportunities and threats (without meaning to sound like a management consultant), and there are several coping strategies that we can employ to help us to live well with very late diagnosis of ASD.

Sarah Hendrickx discusses lifestyle choices for people who have ASD:

> Self-awareness means getting a handle on who you are. Most of us have spent a very long time trying to be somebody else, trying to be acceptable and failing miserably and feeling like an idiot because we 'mess up' all the time and offend people, and nobody quite believes that anyone that bright could be constantly walking on eggshells, waiting until we 'mess things up' the next time. I think it's accepting this reality and saying, 'Yes, that's always going to happen; how can I minimise the damage to myself?' My approach to my own life is pretty bleak, I think, but extraordinarily pragmatic.
>
> I would never say to anyone that it's going to be wonderful, that it's going to be fabulous and you're going to fit in, and it's going to be great. It almost certainly will not be any of those things. What you need to do is not give yourself a hard time and actually just say, 'Okay, you know what? I'm quite awkward in certain situations. I can either avoid those situations or I can learn some strategies and skills to get myself through those situations. No-one – neurotypical or ASD – is great at everything. Some neurotypical people have rubbish social skills and really mess up, too. It's about getting perspective and learning to like yourself.'
>
> I always say to people that my perspective is that we all have a choice, and where you sit on the 'choice line' is your individual decision. You may choose to bend as much as you possibly can: you can try hard to be neurotypical, to fit in, to be nice to

people and so forth. You really can do that if you want, because you're smart enough to do it. You're not going to be entirely fluent, but you'll be reasonably good at it. But you may end up with more mental health problems because it's so exhausting and you're not being true to yourself. The other extreme on that choice line is to be an all-out and outright militant Aspie – walk around being yourself, totally uncompromising, living the world your way. The consequences are that you're unlikely to have a job, relationship and supportive people in your life.

We all need to make our own decision as to where we want to sit on the choice line. It does not have to be all or nothing. There may be a midpoint which allows you to be yourself enough to keep sane and compromise with the neurotypical world enough to get by. That's what I try to do.

If you want all the things that neurotypical people have – jobs, relationships and all that kind of stuff – great! But you're going to have to work really hard to get it. If you want to be yourself, you also have to 'take it on the chin' that you may not get those things because you live in a world where a certain set of rules are required and if you aren't playing the game, you aren't getting the prizes at the end. That's how I see it – that every individual makes their own choice about how much they are willing or able to put in and how much they are willing to accept to get what they want. It's a two-way street. (Sarah Hendrickx, interview, 20 November 2013)

Communication strategies

The following communication strategies are specifically for autistic adults:

- Avoid conflict or confrontation whenever possible, so if disagreement persists, write rather than talk directly, because written words can be toned down later (using filtering procedures) before sending that email or letter.

- Do not communicate with people when you feel angry.

- Never make important decisions hastily or when feeling angry, anxious or depressed.

- For complex communications, it's usually necessary to meet in person or discuss the issue(s) by telephone.

- Avoid important communications when intoxicated or under the influence of any type of drug to decrease the possibility of communicating anything inappropriate or brazenly direct and truthful.

Autistic people are usually better writers than speakers due to our communication difficulties. The following comment was posted on a forum:

> It's very hard for me to talk about my homeless experiences, but I feel it is necessary. I find it much easier and less stressful to write about being homeless than to talk about it. This may in part be due to having PTSD [post-traumatic stress disorder], but it is also an effect of ASD. Writing provides emotional distance and keeps me from getting too overwhelmed by the feelings associated with those times in my life. (Shay 2010)

After diagnosis of ASD, we can prevent misunderstandings by explaining to people that we need others to communicate with us literally and directly because we have difficulty picking up on cues from body language or subtle forms of social etiquette.

Assertiveness training

As mentioned earlier, many people with ASD are easy to manipulate – for several reasons – and often we find it difficult to say 'no'. Also, due to low self-esteem, sometimes we find it difficult to tell people what we really want. Sometimes we are too eager to please others in order to fit in and keep friends, but the main problem is not being able to understand other people's agendas.

A very important keystone of self-empowerment is to honour ourselves and to do what we believe in. Integrity is especially important to autistic people, so we should avoid people who try to corrupt us (or take us away from our 'soul's path') at all costs. This is the main reason why autistic adults should be very discerning about our choice of friends. Remember, we must have purpose, meaning and positive intent to make the world a better place.

If you have an issue with assertiveness, you may consider an assertiveness training workshop, or some one-to-one consultations with a psychologist or psychotherapist. Meanwhile, make friends with people who genuinely respect you and who support you in your endeavours. *Keep away from people who attempt to persuade you to do anything against your will that you know, or even sense, could harm you.*

Selling techniques

I worked as a direct sales representative in London and learned about the principles of selling. These selling techniques are very simple and easy to learn, and they are extremely helpful for survival in a neurotypical world. Understanding these simple neurotypical 'tricks' and applying them to, in effect, sell the positives about our condition to others is bound to eliminate so much struggle from our life. What I am sharing with you here is a set of simple formulas that facilitate our survival in a world where everyone is competing for resources. These techniques, which can be learned quickly, are extremely effective, so they are bound to serve us. Moreover, these simple rules represent a formulaic system that is logical, so every autistic person would benefit from understanding them. I can vouch that this system works for autistic people (as well as for neurotypical people), who, after all, are systemisers.

The Pitney Bowes International sales techniques

Pitney Bowes International taught the following sales techniques (1983):

Sell benefits, not features. A feature is a technical characteristic, such as height, weight, colour or speed. People do not buy products for their features, but for their benefits. When selling, it is essential to translate the product's features into benefits.

For example, a notebook computer may be slim. 'So, what?' the prospective customer may ask. This means that this notebook will benefit users by being light and easy to carry anywhere. Therefore, it would be useful to know whether the prospect likes to work with computers while travelling.

We have two ears and one mouth, and we should use these organs in the same ratio (2:1). When we use our ears effectively, we will identify and log 'buying signals', which are expressions of interest in the product. 'Do you have the notebook in blue?' is a buying signal. If the notebook is available in blue, the salesperson has an opportunity to close the sale if all other potential objections have been overcome. A typical close is, 'If we can provide you with a blue notebook, will you buy it now?'

Always welcome objections! An objection is a reason for not buying the product. For example, 'I don't have enough cash at the moment.' The salesman's job is to log every objection (by listening carefully to the prospect) and then overcome the objections. He may respond, 'So, would you like one month's credit or would you prefer to pay with finance over two years?'

Close the sale when you have overcome all of the customer's objections, when the customer has no reason for not buying the product. There are several closing techniques, including:

- The alternative close, which gives the prospective customer a choice of how to purchase the product. Examples of an alternative close are:
  - 'Would you like to buy the notebook in blue or black?'
  - 'Would you like to buy the notebook with cash or with finance?'
  - 'Do you want to buy this model or that model?'

  When the customer answers with one of the options, they have psychologically committed themselves to buying the product.

- The Wellington close is a heavyweight closing technique: If I can overcome (your specified objections) will you buy the

> product? For example, 'If I could provide the product in blue and arrange finance for you, would you purchase the product now?'

How would this relate to 'selling' yourself? Well, sales techniques can help us get whatever we want in any areas of life, whether it's a job, a business appointment, a research grant or a date.

Anger management

Anger disturbs our well-being, so everyone is best advised to eliminate any feelings of anger, hate and revenge as soon as possible. Autistic adults – particularly during the post-diagnostic identity crisis – probably have more reasons for being angry than most people, especially those of us who have been abused, bullied, cheated or otherwise exploited.

As emphasised in, for example, the principles of Twelve-Step programmes (such as Alcoholics Anonymous), which are used by addiction support groups worldwide, we need to forgive *ourselves* first and foremost, and need to cut all emotional involvement with people who do not have our best interests at heart. In order to take full responsibility for ourselves, we need to *forgive ourselves for allowing others to mistreat us.*

As mentioned under 'Communication strategies', autistic individuals are usually unable to cope with conflict, so we should avoid communication when we feel angry, bitter or resentful.

Self-identification of our mental condition, and finally understanding why we have always been treated differently, certainly helps to defuse the anger. Now we understand that people who did not understand *us*, and perhaps mistreated us, were simply being their neurotypical selves while we were being our autistic selves.

Relaxation

The most effective way for autistic people to relax is to pursue our special interests with as much focus and passion as possible. The great news is that we are tuned into our special interests, so we don't need anyone else to advise us on what to do!

Writing is therapeutic, and we may benefit from maintaining a personal journal (keep it going beyond the post-diagnostic crisis) to record insights and lessons. Also, consider establishing a regular online blog to share your knowledge with others, or write a book about your special interest.

Some autistic people derive benefit from meditation and mindfulness techniques, while others enjoy playing with words (wordplay) or numbers (numberplay).

Playing with words and numbers

An example of wordplay is:

> Eleven was a racehorse
> Twelve was one two
> Eleven won one race
> Twelve won one too.

This riddle (whose author is anonymous) may also be expressed using numberplay as follows:

> 11 was a racehorse
> 12 was 12
> 11 11 race
> 12 112.

Getting healthy exercise in beautiful, natural environments is also a way to relax. A strong cardiovascular workout – ideally by cross-country running, cycling or similar activities – is recommended. These forms of exercise, which can be performed alone or with a friend, will also facilitate deeper sleep. Travelling to new places of interest or foreign cultures is another exciting and educational way to unwind. Also uplifting and relaxing is riding a motorcycle or bicycle through beautiful countryside. Because we are ungrounded and often locked inside our intellectual bubble, we benefit from all kinds of physical activities (others are dance, massage, yoga, tai chi and martial arts). Spending time in nature also supports our healing process, so activities such as gardening, hiking and travel photography are highly recommended.

Getting support

After self-identification or diagnosis we have many needs, so these support services may be necessary to get us on the right track:

- mentoring to understand ourselves better and become clear about our gifts and deficits

- coaching to support our attainment of specific goals, such as getting a job, dating, withdrawing from substances or starting a business

- facilitated ASD support groups and person-centred facilitation to empower us, address our needs and improve our quality of life

- counselling or psychotherapy to help resolve painful issues, reach closure with unhealthy relationships and/or change the way we perceive ourselves.

Inappropriate support by practitioners who lack knowledge about ASD can be harmful. Be aware that most counsellors and psychotherapists are trained to consult neurotypical people only. The autistic mind is different, so support workers must have extensive knowledge about ASD.

Few recently diagnosed adults are likely to have sufficient resources available to address all the above needs (in addition to psychological assessment and diagnosis, which may be a challenge alone). Although there are many practitioners who claim to specialise in autism, the top tier of autism professionals are extremely expensive.

There are many fantastic ASD forums where you can socialise and get support from fellow Aspies. Find out from these people what strategies they used because their ideas might work for you. Try to get help if you need support, and find an interest and reward yourself every now and then. I found Toastmasters (www.toastmasters.org) to be a fantastic place to learn communication and social skills. Also consider relaxation exercises. (Roderick Wintour, correspondence, 10 December 2013)

Mentoring

Mentoring is a long-term relationship that meets a development need, helps develop full potential and benefits all partners including the mentor, mentee and organisation. (Suzanne Faure, cited in Gibbons 1999)

People who have ASD usually need a mentor after self-identification, until they have fully accepted themselves. The mentor should be a fully integrated person with ASD or a full-time autism practitioner who is genuinely empathetic towards ASD culture. The purpose of the ASD mentor is to guide us towards self-acceptance and a fulfilling, independent life. The mentor should also empower us by making us aware of our gifts as well as our impairments. The ASD mentoring can be conducted face to face or by telephone, Skype or email. Some mentors charge on an hourly basis, while others offer their service on a donation-only basis.

The mentor should normally provide a *long-term* supportive relationship because the process of identity alignment (between self-identification and self-acceptance) can take several years, and some autistic people never make peace with themselves as people who have ASD because 'it is widely perceived as a neurological and developmental problem and they cannot or will not acknowledge that they have this disability', says Sara Heath.

The role of the ASD mentor is to support us to come to terms with the difficulties and problems that having ASD causes, to learn to accept the past and look towards the future, to translate and explain issues into our own contexts of experience, to clarify difficult concepts to aid understanding, to explore strengths and weaknesses and to empower the client to work through his or her issues to facilitate a more positive and rewarding life. (Sara Heath, correspondence, 13 November 2013)

Tony Attwood compares a recently self-identified autistic adult without a mentor (or similar support) to a boat without a rudder.

Coaching

Coaches help us to achieve specific goals, which may involve lifestyle change, or career, financial or relationship goals. Specifically, a coach may help an autistic person to achieve any of the following goals:

- get a job
- find a relationship partner
- become financially independent
- live autonomously
- learn a new skill.

Life coaching usually aims to transform a client's lifestyle and improve his or her quality of life. The main value to the person with ASD lies in the executive planning and strategy (or project management) which is usually challenging for us.

The ASD coach Bill Goodyear states:

Coaching is essentially a dialogue between two people, it is fuelled by some deep understandings and ways of thinking that allow the coach to build up a beneficial influence, although it is the subjects of the coaching who have to do all the hard work and make the changes in the way they experience their lives. (Goodyear 2008, p.xiv)

Autistic people experience the world in a very different way, and it is this experience that damages us so much. We learn to be different because we are excluded, which magnifies the original condition. We learn negative thinking in response to repeated negative experiences.

Home life

Autistic adults have extremely diverse lifestyles. Sara Heath states:

> We are talking about people over forty here. Some parents have died; some are estranged from parents but still see them occasionally at the shops or in the area; some live with parents; some are cared for by parents; some are married and are cared for by wife or husband; some are single with no carers; some are cared for by children or a paid carer; and many have parents who are elderly and could be caring for them! (Sara Heath, correspondence, 17 February 2013)

Anyone who has autism may benefit from living in a foreign country because people from other cultures may be less aware of our differences. (Expats, whether strong or disabled, are generally treated with respect in Southeast Asia, as long as we respect the local culture and customs – and pay our bills, of course!)

> Very few people with Asperger syndrome (ASD) venture far from home, but there are massive benefits of living in a foreign culture. Very often our differences are not looked upon with so much disdain in another culture. 'He's a foreigner! That's why he is different!' they say. So, you are given more of a 'behavioural pass' in another culture. One way to escape the negative judgements that arise from bigotry and stigmas is therefore to live overseas. (Michael John Carley, interview, 16 November 2012)

Similarly, Altazar Rossiter recognises the benefits of living overseas:

> I also think that living outside the UK (disconnected from the debilitating cultural matrix you learned to define yourself within) will have helped you in coming to understand yourself better. I know you've always questioned the insanity you experienced here. That particular brand of insanity is called 'Englishness'. It is an energy matrix that defined your existence as you learned to make an identity for yourself. It's not necessarily better or worse than any other, but living outside it enables a clearer perception of it. (Altazar Rossiter, correspondence, 29 November 2012)

My experience of living in Thailand

I began a new life in Chiang Mai in February 2003 and lived for seven years in the same guesthouse. In those days, the Thais were especially kind and welcoming, so I felt like a member of a royal family. By contrast, in England I felt depressed because people projected their negative images onto me and my sensitive nature would easily absorb their negative thoughts. However, when I arrived in Thailand – known as 'The Land of Smiles' – I was welcomed by the warm, open-hearted Thai people. I sometimes wonder whether I would have identified my condition if I had stayed in England – and, indeed, whether I would be alive right now.

Autistic people are naturally independent individuals, so even if living abroad isn't a realistic solution, it is still crucial to find an ideal home environment which is suitable or which we can adapt to our needs. For instance, many autistic people believe in sustainable living; therefore, an ideal place for many nature-loving autistic people could be a farm that utilises renewable energy and has access to its own natural water and food supplies.

The ideal place to live for some autistic adults is one that is free of all forms of pollution. People with ASD are vulnerable to sensory overload, so it is important that we live in a serene place that supports a relaxed lifestyle. Everyone can improve their quality of life by eating fresh, organic produce and drinking fresh water in a clean, natural environment that is free of pollution.

Nature's healing power

Nature is a healing power for people with ASD and is the best recipe for mental health. I believe that autistic people are natural healers and shamans. In one of the documentaries on the Wrong Planet website, Alex Plank interviewed a shaman, Dr Edward Hall, who said that autistic people are suited to the Red Path of shamanism (Plank 2009). Our cultural style is slower and more profound than neurotypical culture, so we are able to conceive things on an energetic level rather than being limited to scientific reality. Autism is about simplification and breaking things down to the essentials, so the key to our well-being is unity with nature. The words 'sustainability' and 'self-sufficiency' are key to peace of mind.

So what is the most autism-friendly country in the world? The wrongplanet.net forum cites Wales (UK) as a supportive place for autistic people. If we go to the other side of the world, in New Zealand, support services for ASD have traditionally been left to volunteers; the official thinking generally is 'Let the volunteers keep doing it!' Also, because New Zealand is a small country with a limited number of taxpayers, it cannot afford to support all health and medical-related support organisations. But this is no bad thing. Jen Birch states:

> I believe that New Zealand has an influential culture of ordinary people taking on voluntary roles in charitable organisations. Autism New Zealand is in the category of minimal government support, and whatever financial support there was a few years ago is gradually being taken away due to financial cuts. But Autism New Zealand (and other similar organisations in the country) do a good job on a financial shoestring of providing information, guidance, moral support, training courses and support groups to its members and enquirers. (Jen Birch, correspondence, 26 November 2012)

> I think the UK is probably one of the best countries in the world for autistic people; not that the UK is good, but actually everywhere else is worse. I'm not aware of any country where more or better support is available, except perhaps Holland and Scandinavian countries. (Sarah Hendrickx, interview, 20 November 2013)

The Auckland Branch of Autism New Zealand provides an adult AS social group (with two get-togethers every month), an Asperger youth group, an Asperger women's group and various other support groups and training courses for parents, training seminars for teaching staff, free phone and email helplines, regular newsletters, a national conference every two years and a bookstore for ASD books, DVDs and other AS-related resources. Currently, Autism New Zealand has some paid staff as well as many volunteers in various roles, so although New Zealand does not offer much financial support to Aspies, there is support available among the not-for-profit organisations and groups – which brings us to the subject of making sure we have adequate financial resources (Jen Birch, correspondence, 26 November 2012).

Money

Researchers at the Carnegie Institute of Technology in the US report that 85 per cent of our financial success depends upon our personality, as well as communication, negotiation and leadership skills, while just 15 per cent of financial success is due to technical knowledge (Jensen 2012). Naturally, this places autistic people at a massive disadvantage.

In a corporate environment, the most respected people are confident, well presented, socially adept communicators. The 'winners' are savvy with social etiquette, understand unwritten rules, are empathetic and relate well with higher authorities.

In the past, a high intelligence quotient and hard work were sufficient to guarantee financial success, but now our emotional intelligence or quotient (EQ) and moral quotient (MQ) are similarly important prerequisites for success. Our EQ enables us to be aware of our own and others' feelings while managing our emotions and building sustainable relationships. Our MQ concerns our integrity, reliability and responsibility (Jensen 2012).

Autistic people tend to have low EQ because we lack cognitive empathy, which is the ability to perceive other people's thoughts and feelings, so we find it difficult to sustain relationships. The MQ is more complex because, although people who have ASD can be fixated on the truth, and we are usually on time for appointments and meet important deadlines, our 'different' behaviour often causes people to judge us as irresponsible and unreliable.

Here are some ideas about how we can improve our relationship with money:

- Record income and expenses, make budgets and forecasts, and attempt to understand which costs are essential and which are not.

- Find out exactly how much money you need and then ask appropriate people to help you access it.

- Avoid debt and bank fees, if possible.

- Try to create royalty-based income streams from your creative projects.

- Remember that the best investments are in yourself! Invest in your quality of life and self-improvement, rather than simply following fashion.

Find appropriate work

Our 'impairments' have been publicised everywhere from general interest magazines to specialist publications including the APA's *DSM-5*. While it's good to be aware of our weaknesses, it's important to be positive and clear – for ourselves and employers – about our strengths and 'gifts'.

The main positive characteristics of autistic people are:

- *Original thinking:* People with ASD have the ability to think outside the box because the 'box' limits us with its social and unwritten rules and customs. Autistic people are less inhibited by cultural and social restrictions and are therefore able to apply logic without such limitations.

- *Protracted focus:* Autistic people are able to focus attention on tasks for long periods of time when the tasks are meaningful or related to a special interest.

- *Systemising ability:* People with ASD are highly logical with adept ability to perceive relationships between people, objects, systems, time and space.

- *Truthfulness and sense of justice:* Autistic people are compelled to seek truth and justice, and to express it to others.

- *Abstract thinking:* People with ASD have high ability to generate abstract ideas during 'brainstorming' sessions.

- *Connection with nature:* Most autistic people are peaceful people who enjoy nature and animals.

- *Ability to simplify complex issues:* People with ASD have a unique ability to understand large quantities of complex and disparate information and draw clear, simple conclusions.

- *Attention to detail:* Autistic people are able to quickly learn detailed routines and patterns in data sets, and to notice errors easily.

- *Multidimensional thinking:* People with ASD are able to think in ways that neurotypical people cannot, and can often identify solutions that neurotypical people find difficult, or even impossible, to understand.

Read and re-read this list of autistic strengths, believe them and tell everyone about them. Add other 'gifts' to this list. This practice helps us to increase our confidence.

For an autistic person's job to be sustainable, the following prerequisites apply:

- The work must be meaningful, purposeful and interesting.

- We must be allowed 'ownership' and control over how we carry out our job.

- The work environment needs to be relaxing, not too noisy and free of bullying, herd mentality and discriminatory office politics.

- We need to have access to empathetic, supportive co-workers and bosses.

Remember that we are most productive when we feel comfortable and relaxed, and free of annoying disturbances. For example, it is better for us to work in a clean room containing natural light and fresh air, preferably with an inspiring view. There should be minimal clutter and background noise. Some people like to have their pet around them at all times, too. The following jobs are potentially suitable for adults who have ASD:

- radio deejay

- cartographer

- dentist

- proofreader

- editor

- computer programmer

- gardener

- librarian

- facilitator (in an area of special interest)

- market researcher

- shaman

- business analyst.

Although some autistic adults survive in the following jobs, many don't because they demand adept social, communication, multitasking and executive skills:

- politician

- advertising executive

- beauty consultant

- project manager

- human resources manager

- TV presenter.

Here are some tips about how to find appropriate employment:

- Focus on your strengths instead of weaknesses and memorise your personal list of 'unique selling points' that will convince the employer that *you* are the ideal candidate for the job.

- Register with inclusive recruitment consultants, such as Evenbreak (www.evenbreak.co.uk), who promote accommodations in the workforce for disabled people.

- Apply for jobs with organisations that are actively seeking talented and motivated people on the autism spectrum, such as SAP International.

- Use online professional networking platforms, such as LinkedIn and Twitter, to source appropriate human resource managers and inclusive recruiters.

- Hire a coach who is knowledgeable about ASD to help with the job-seeking process.

    One little strategy that I use which has won me several jobs is to ask for a job interview in a few days time, and then to volunteer my services free of charge before the interview. This means that the employer is already aware of my capabilities by the time of the interview. Employers love it! (Roderick Wintour, correspondence, 10 December 2013)

Love and relationships

Being in a healthy relationship with a compassionate and patient person who is willing to learn about ASD is probably the best form of support. On the other hand, being in an inappropriate relationship with an abusive or controlling person can make our situation much worse. Be aware that there is a very powerful law of attraction between similar people who have neurological conditions. Moreover, there is an equally strong attraction between opposite personality types – for example, autistic people (who cannot perceive other peoples' intentions) and abusive people who lack affective empathy. Other types who love to attach onto vulnerable autistic people are control freaks and people who use other people to enable themselves to feel better.

There are several reasons why people on the autism spectrum have relationship problems, but one of the key issues is lack of theory of mind (or cognitive empathy).

> Another issue is that people with more classic autism are often happy in their own bubbles, do not miss the attachment and do not care what others think of them. They do not need to wear a social mask – they are the way they are. However, other people with ASD are in their bubbles looking out and wanting to be in the world, but as they are 'aliens' they do not have a manual and have to learn as they go along. They want others to think well of them, so they put on a social mask and pretend that they are not who they really are – and this exhausts them. The breakdown often occurs when the mask slips off and the real ASD person is revealed, 'warts and all' – and this can tip them over the edge into depression and self-harm. (Sara Heath, correspondence, 17 February 2013)

There are potentially five different types of love in an autistic person's life:

1. Secure attachment during the infant's development which, as mentioned earlier, is described by Simon Baron-Cohen as 'the internal pot of gold'.

2. Passion for special interests and pride in meaningful projects ('Aspie love').

3. Unconditional familial love from parents, siblings and other relatives who offer love and support without question, thus providing a safety blanket for when situations go awry.

4. Genuinely supportive friends who help us to achieve what we really want.

5. A caring relationship partner for intimacy and sexual fulfilment.

Autistic people are normally visual thinkers, so we can access our memory like rewinding a video; therefore, visual arts, such as photography and video production, can be extremely fulfilling for many of us. Moreover, proximity to nature and contact with animals has a therapeutic effect on us, so gardening and other outdoor pursuits are also recommended.

Passion for special interests

Most adults who have ASD follow their passion for special interests and meaningful work. This passion may be a replacement for the love that most normal people receive. The area of interest may be extremely narrow and offbeat. As Michael Fitzgerald notes, some autistic people achieve fame or notoriety during their lifetime (e.g. Mozart and Einstein), while many others are only acknowledged posthumously (interview, 10 October 2013).

Passion for special interests is the autistic love that brings meaningfulness to our lives. Most neurotypical people do not value this form of love as much as we do; instead, they prefer relationship partners (often in structured relationship contracts, such as marriage), strong family bonds, business contacts and a good social life.

Unconditional familial love

Autistic adults often lack access to unconditional familial love; this explains why we need security and routines to feel safe. Many mature adults who have ASD do not have any parents or carers, and many of our parents could not accept us for being 'different', so we lack a familial safety net to support us during hard times.

A female shaman said that if all couples conceived their children in an atmosphere of unconditional love, there would not be any trouble in this world.

Genuinely supportive friends

It is more difficult for autistic people to develop a circle of genuinely supportive friends because we are poor judges of character. Also, because people with ASD tend to be introverted and lacking in self-esteem and assertiveness, others tend to choose us as their friends rather than the other way around. So the way to turn things around is to be discerning, screen potential friends for abusive characteristics and be proud of our strengths.

> I think the more that people immerse themselves into some kind of autistic community – whether that be a group, reading online, watching videos of people with autism sharing their experiences and so forth – the greater that benefit is, because there is comfort in knowing that you're not alone. There is comfort in reading or hearing or speaking to somebody and thinking, *That's how it is for me, but nobody else gets it.* It's very helpful to feel accepted. I wonder if self-acceptance can be separated from some kind of societal acceptance or acceptance by a significant other, because I think that's quite important. You need other relationships to support self-acceptance. It's very difficult to be totally self-accepting if you are totally on your own.
>
> If you're continuing to get negative feedback from the outside world that says, 'You're rude. You're weird. You don't fit in,' you would have to be a rhino-headed individual to completely and utterly disregard these judgements. I think most people might say, 'I don't care what anybody thinks of me,' but actually most of us do care to a degree. So acceptance from others, I think, is crucial in self-acceptance. You feel that you're getting it right somewhere in the world with someone, even if it's only one person. (Sarah Hendrickx, interview, 20 November 2013)

A caring relationship partner

Many autistic adults give up on relationships after several disastrous encounters. The chance of the relationship being successful is slim if we have not yet identified our condition.

Also, a neurotypical relationship partner needs to be extremely tolerant and understanding for the relationship to survive so many misunderstandings and arguments.

Maxine Aston's relationship tips for people on the spectrum

- If you are already in a relationship, don't discontinue it just because you are (and/or your partner is) on the autism spectrum. Asperger syndrome (ASD) should not be judged as either good or bad; however, for a relationship to be successful, both parties need to have compatible personalities. The success or failure of the relationship does not depend upon the neurological condition of either partner, but instead on the compatibility of their personalities, values, goals and interests, commitment to the relationship and whether they really care.

- If your relationship partner 'blows up' with temper tantrums because he or she cannot accept your autistic limitations (such as not being able to identify emotional cues), they need to understand that this behaviour is unacceptable. The ASD will never go away, so if your partner cannot accept this fact, it's better to break up the relationship. Typically, in these situations the autistic men are passive and quiet, while their neurotypical partners can be volatile and oppressive with their own emotional issues.

- An increasing number of autistic adults are seeking foreign relationship partners using the Internet. Having cross-cultural relationships can disguise communication difficulties because both people are from different cultures, so misunderstandings are often excused initially; however, Maxine says that this strategy works only for a while.

- Being in an inappropriate relationship can cause misery, so if relationship issues cannot be resolved, it is usually best to end it. Being single or alone is preferable to being in an unbalanced relationship that causes undue suffering.

- Autistic people tend to focus on peoples' mouths instead of their eyes when we communicate. We see the smile which is a sign of friendliness, kindness or even a sign of attraction. We are not able to identify the glimmer in the eyes that says, 'Hey, I'm getting out of here!' So try to look at the person's eyes instead of their mouth to pick up more communication signals, or try to get someone else's opinion.

- People who are on the autism spectrum require less frequent relationship counselling than neurotypical people because our minds process information much slower and need longer time to reflect. Typically, Maxine provides just one or two counselling sessions each month to people who have ASD.

- Never compromise who you are. 'If you start to compromise the essence of who you are, you will lose yourself and your self-esteem. If the other person cannot accept you for who you are, then they're not the person you need to be with.'

- A question that many autistic people ask Maxine is, 'Does he (or she) really like me?' Maxine recommends that we pay more attention to their behaviour. 'Don't go by what they say or promise, so forget the words!' Instead, we should try to notice what they are actually doing to show that they genuinely care about us.

- Do not commit too quickly because the test of time is a good filter for relationships.

Another matter to consider is that most adults with ASD also have poor mental health, and most have anxiety and depression, which creates an invisible barrier between lovers. Mental ill health and medication tend to impair sex drive, and autistic people have a lower threshold to sensual overload.

Probably less than 33 per cent of Aspergic adults are in a relationship, and many of their partners are from foreign cultures

(Wylie and Heath 2013). Neurotypical people who are not from an autistic person's native country are less likely to perceive the autistic person as abnormal, so many of us have cross-cultural relationships.

> Men with Asperger syndrome who are in a relationship with a neurotypical woman who is on the opposite end of the empathy scale, such as counsellors, psychotherapists, nurses, teachers and other generally nurturing people, usually struggle to meet their partner's very high emotional needs. These women can often place unrealistic emotional demands on their partners. This has happened in almost every Aspie/neurotypical relationship that I've seen in the couples that have come to me for support. I often ask my clients to do the Empathy Quotient (EQ) test just to show them how far apart they are on the EQ scale. They are on the extremes: whereas the average is somewhere in the 40s, she scores 75 and he scores 6. This is a common pattern that I see.
>
> In my experience, Aspie relationships with other Aspies work better than mixed (i.e. Aspie–neurotypical) relationships. The majority of people with ASD that I know socially have partners that are either diagnosed or could be diagnosed, so they're in a relationship with somebody pretty similar in terms of neurological profile. It seems to work. (I can't see why it *wouldn't* work.) My partner and I live almost in parallel to each other without that enormous intuitive emotional expectation that if I'm wandering around the kitchen banging saucepans, he's going to actually know what that means and therefore what he needs to do about it. We don't do that. I just say, 'I'm pissed off, and it's because of this. I need you to do this,' and he says, 'Okay, I'll do that.' Problem solved. There's no sulking. There's no 'Couldn't you tell I was upset?' We just don't bother because we know that those signals are not going to be picked up. It's just so much more straightforward. Our relationship is based on two people looking for practical solutions and who want to be happy. You tell me there's a problem and I'll try to fix it.

That's it! It's bliss. (Sarah Hendrickx, interview, 20 November 2013)

The APA provides a free interactive online test to assess your current relationship (see http://allpsych.com/tests/self-help/relationship. html). You will receive the result immediately after answering ten simple questions. Also, an excellent book about making an Asperger marriage work is that by Katrin Bentley (2007) with contributions from her husband, who has ASD.

A lot of people with Asperger syndrome have very strong qualities for a loving relationship, but the main thing to remember is that the outcome of romantic relationships depends on how much effort both parties put into the relationship, because it's not a one-way street. Make sure that your partner knows what to expect and be very honest with them about that. Have no secrets and be a giver and not a taker. Be willing to make sacrifices, such as confronting a fear of being unsociable, so that your partner is not deprived of that experience. Love will give you the strength; if it doesn't, you're not in love. (Roderick Wintour, correspondence, 10 December 2013)

Health

Natural health remedies, and alternative and complementary medicines, are favoured by many adults who have ASD. We prefer natural solutions to synthetic ones, and many of us have a deep distrust of psychiatry, which classifies ASD as a disorder. Popular natural remedies for autistic people are melatonin and valerian (to promote sound sleep) and St John's wort (to reduce depression), as well as multivitamins.

Many autistic adults prefer not to have contact with doctors, so when the need arises, they might self-medicate using alcohol and/ or other substances.

Drinking and substance misuse can also be due to not getting the right help, support, understanding, jobs and relationships, and is a constant when life is not comfortable. It works as a social lubricant, so it helps with these issues – it breaks the ice and reduces the innate inhibitions related to ASD – and alcohol is legal. Sarah Hendrickx wrote a good book [see Hendrickx and Tinsley 2008 in Further Reading] about ASD and alcohol, so again it is not only attachment issues that lead ASD people to drink – drink can help with social issues and stress reduction, and many people with ASD will not see a general practitioner and will never have mental health support – it's self-medication. (Sara Heath, correspondence, 17 February 2013)

Regular exercise is an effective way of combating mental illness and uplifting our spirits. When we exercise, our brain releases endorphins, which enables us to relax.

Lifestyle

Autistic adults are suited to quiet, natural environments, so many autistic people (including Temple Grandin) work with animals on farms. Nature is the best healer.

Shamanic work, in my understanding, is about making your own personal and unique relationship with the universe and the natural energies of everything in existence. It's about recognising our connection with all there is and making our own meaning. Aspergic people may well be suited for shamanic work in a way that may more easily create for them a structured relationship with the universe that has no connection with the conventions of their culture. Their existence in this world of their own definition and their conflict with consensus paradigms may seem perfectly ordinary, so they are better able to function outside convention. (Altazar Rossiter, correspondence, 29 November 2012)

Some final words

On a cautionary note, Luke Beardon states:

Be extremely careful what you read and who you listen to, because much of what is written and discussed in relation to

ASD is inaccurate. Even the best writing about ASD is not completely relevant to all individuals. Post-diagnostic support is crucial, so be very careful about where it comes from! (Luke Beardon, correspondence, 31 January 2013)

On a positive note, here are my top ten survival tips for a more fulfilling future:

1. Whenever possible, stick with natural medicine, physical exercise and other empowering panaceas as alternatives to formal or institutional health care.

2. Consider freelance work, particularly royalty-based projects, or voluntary work as a means to financial independence and personal fulfilment.

3. Follow your passion always and maintain positive intent to serve humanity.

4. Be selective about your friends and who you confide in about your condition.

5. Analyse your family psychological history to identify the genetic path of autism and other psychiatric conditions in your family, because this vital knowledge supports self-understanding and forgiveness.

6. Use a mentor during your crisis – online, if necessary – and consider maintaining a journal as well; and use an ASD coach to help you reach your goals.

7. Consult full-time autism practitioners only (ideally those who have ASD).

8. Forget about 'cures' for ASD because there aren't any, and we don't need them (but we do need tolerance of neurodiversity).

9. Consider living in another country, culture or environment to avoid mistreatment.

10. Above all, focus on the light at the end of the tunnel!

INTERNATIONAL DIRECTORY OF RESOURCES

Name of Organisation	Location	Website Address	Further Information
Advocacy and Information			
Australian Advisory Board on Autism Spectrum Disorders (AABASD)	Australia	www.autismaus.com.au	AABASD is Australia's umbrella organisation for autism.
Autism Association of Western Australia	Australia	www.autism.org.au	The Autism Association of Western Australia is a member of AABASD.
Autism Europe	Europe	www.autismeurope.org	Autism Europe is based in Belgium.
Autism New Zealand Inc.	New Zealand	www.autismnz.org.nz	Autism New Zealand Inc. provides support, training, advocacy, resources and information about the autism spectrum.
Autism Queensland	Australia	www.autismqld.com.au	Autism Queensland Inc. is a member of AABASD.
Autism Society of America (ASOA)	USA	www.autism-society.org	ASOA provides advocacy, information and research for autistic people, their families and carers.

Autism Society Canada (ASC)	Canada	www.autismsocietycanada.ca	ASC is a federation of Canada-wide provincial and territorial autism societies.
Autism Southern Australia (Autism SA)	Australia	www.autismsa.org.au	Autism SA is a member of AABASD.
Autism Speaks	USA	www.autismspeaks.org	Autism Speaks provides information and advocacy for autistic people.
Autism Spectrum Australia (Aspect)	Australia	www.autismspectrum.org.au	Aspect is a member of AABASD.
Autism Tasmania	Australia	www.autismtas.org.au	Autism Tasmania is a member of AABASD.
Autism Victoria (Amaze)	Australia	www.autismvictoria.org.au/home	Amaze is a member of AABASD.
National Autistic Society (NAS)	UK	www.nas.org.uk	NAS is the leading UK charity for people with autism (including Asperger syndrome) and their families. The charity provides information, support and professional services, and campaigns for a better world for people with autism.
Neurodiversity.com	Internet	www.neurodiversity.com/main.html	Neurodiversity.com provides comprehensive information resources.
Online Asperger Syndrome Information & Support (OASIS)	USA	www.aspergersyndrome.org	OASIS offers information and advocacy for families and individuals.

Conferences and Exhibitions

Autism Conferences of America, LLC (ACA)	USA	www. autismconferencesofamerica. com	ACA is an approved California Regional Center vendor.
Autism New Zealand Inc. conference	New Zealand	www.autismnz.org.nz/ about_us/conference_2012	
The Autism Show	UK	www.autismshow.co.uk	The Autism Show is hosted in both London and Manchester.
Irish Society for Autism	Ireland	www.autism.ie	The 2013 conference was held in Dublin.
National Autistic Society's Professional Conference	UK	www.autism.org.uk/ news-and-events/nas-conference.aspx	The Professional Conference is about current best practices for senior autism practitioners.

Internet Blogs and Forums

Neurodiversity weblog	Internet	www.neurodiversity.com	Information, news, letters and announcements
Shift Journal	Internet	www.shiftjournal.com	Shift Journal is about autism, neurodiversity and social change.
Wrong Planet	Internet	www.wrongplanet.net	Wrong Planet offers discussions on all aspects of the autism spectrum.

Lawyers for Autism

Lawyers.com	USA	www.lawyers.com/Autism/ browse-by-location.html	Autism lawyers by US state.

Magazines

Asperger United	UK	www.autism.org.uk/aspergerunited	Asperger United is the quarterly magazine of the National Autistic Society.
Autism Asperger's Digest	USA	autismdigest.com	Quarterly magazine available in print as well as digital app for Apple iOS and ebook in PDF format.
Autism Spectrum Quarterly	Internet	www.asquarterly.com	ASQ is a quarterly online magazine based in the USA.
British Journal of Psychiatry	UK	bjp.rcpsych.org	

Online Assessment

The AQ Test	Internet	www.wired.com/wired/archive/9.12/aqtest.html	This test for AS contains 50 online questions.
Autism Research Centre (ARC), Cambridge University	UK	www.autismresearchcentre.com/arc_tests	The ARC website provides downloadable tests for research purposes only.

Pre-diagnostic Assessments

Autonomy	UK and International	www.shropshireautonomy.co.uk	Autonomy provides local support groups, training, and both pre- and post-diagnostic assessments.

Psychiatry

American Psychiatric Association (APA)	USA	www.psychiatry.org/network	The APA website provides a searchable database of psychiatrists.
APA's DSM-5 Development website	USA	www.dsm5.org	Information on the fifth edition of the *Diagnostic and Statistical Manual of Mental Disorders*.
Royal College of Psychiatrists	UK	www.rcpsych.ac.uk	

Publications			
Autism Speaks (Apps)	Internet	www.autismspeaks.org/autism-apps	Autism-related apps for iPads, iPhone, iTouch and Android.
Jessica Kingsley Publishers (JKP)	International	www.jkp.com	JKP publishes specialist books for the autism community.
Research			
Autism Research Centre (ARC), Cambridge University	UK	www.autismresearchcentre.com	ARC accepts NHS referrals for diagnosis of autistic adults.
Autistica	UK	www.autistica.org.uk	Autistica is a registered charity for the research into the causes of AS.
Interactive Autism Network (IAN)	USA	www.iancommunity.org	IAN Research is an online longitudinal database and research registry. Families and affected individuals throughout the US share their information with autism researchers and are notified about studies for which they qualify.
Research Autism UK	UK	www.researchautism.net	Research Autism is a UK research charity.
Support Groups			
GRASP	USA and Canada	www.grasp.org	GRASP provides a network of facilitated autism support groups across America and Canada.
National Autism Association	USA	www.nationalautismassociation.org	
Training Courses			
Hendrickx Associates	UK	www.asperger-training.com	Sarah Hendrickx provides training workshops about Asperger syndrome, as well as assessments and consultancy.

Appendix

THE ADULT AUTISM SPECTRUM QUOTIENT (AQ)

AGES 16+: SCORING KEY

For full details, please see: S. Baron-Cohen, S. Wheelwright, R. Skinner, J. Martin and E. Clubley (2001), 'The Autism Spectrum Quotient (AQ): Evidence from Asperger Syndrome/High Functioning Autism, males and females, scientists and mathematicians,' *Journal of Autism and Developmental Disorders 31*, 5–17.

The Autism Spectrum Quotient (AQ) is provided 'as is' and the creators, Professor Simon Baron-Cohen and Sally Wheelwright, the Autism Research Centre and the University of Cambridge, make no warranties of any kind, either express or implied, concerning the AQ. The AQ is provided for research use only and should not be used to inform clinical decisions. Any commercial use of the AQ is prohibited without prior express written permission from the creators and the Autism Research Centre at the University of Cambridge.

Responses that score 1 point are marked. Other responses score 0. For total score, sum all items.

		definitely agree	slightly agree	slightly disagree	definitely disagree
1.	I prefer to do things with others rather than on my own.			1	1
2.	I prefer to do things the same way over and over again.	1	1		
3.	If I try to imagine something, I find it very easy to create a picture in my mind.			1	1
4.	I frequently get so strongly absorbed in one thing that I lose sight of other things.	1	1		

5.	I often notice small sounds when others do not.	1	1		
6.	I usually notice car number plates or similar strings of information.	1	1		
7.	Other people frequently tell me that what I've said is impolite, even though I think it is polite.	1	1		
8.	When I'm reading a story, I can easily imagine what the characters might look like.			1	1
9.	I am fascinated by dates.	1	1		
10.	In a social group, I can easily keep track of several different people's conversations.			1	1
11.	I find social situations easy.			1	1
12.	I tend to notice details that others do not.	1	1		
13.	I would rather go to a library than to a party.	1	1		
14.	I find making up stories easy.			1	1
15.	I find myself drawn more strongly to people than to things.			1	1
16.	I tend to have very strong interests, which I get upset about if I can't pursue.	1	1		
17.	I enjoy social chitchat.			1	1
18.	When I talk, it isn't always easy for others to get a word in edgeways.	1	1		
19.	I am fascinated by numbers.	1	1		
20.	When I'm reading a story, I find it difficult to work out the characters' intentions.	1	1		

21. I don't particularly enjoy reading fiction.	1	1		
22. I find it hard to make new friends.	1	1		
23. I notice patterns in things all the time.	1	1		
24. I would rather go to the theatre than to a museum.			1	1
25. It does not upset me if my daily routine is disturbed.			1	1
26. I frequently find that I don't know how to keep a conversation going.	1	1		
27. I find it easy to 'read between the lines' when someone is talking to me.			1	1
28. I usually concentrate more on the whole picture, rather than on the small details.			1	1
29. I am not very good at remembering phone numbers.			1	1
30. I don't usually notice small changes in a situation, or a person's appearance.			1	1
31. I know how to tell if someone listening to me is getting bored.			1	1
32. I find it easy to do more than one thing at once.			1	1
33. When I talk on the phone, I'm not sure when it's my turn to speak.	1	1		
34. I enjoy doing things spontaneously.			1	1
35. I am often the last to understand the point of a joke.	1	1		

36. I find it easy to work out what someone is thinking or feeling just by looking at their face.			1	1
37. If there is an interruption, I can switch back to what I was doing very quickly.			1	1
38. I am good at social chitchat.			1	1
39. People often tell me that I keep going on and on about the same thing.	1	1		
40. When I was young, I used to enjoy playing games involving pretending with other children.			1	1
41. I like to collect information about categories of things (e.g. types of cars, birds, trains, plants).	1	1		
42. I find it difficult to imagine what it would be like to be someone else.	1	1		
43. I like to carefully plan any activities I participate in.	1	1		
44. I enjoy social occasions.			1	1
45. I find it difficult to work out people's intentions.	1	1		
46. New situations make me anxious.	1	1		
47. I enjoy meeting new people.			1	1
48. I am a good diplomat.			1	1
49. I am not very good at remembering people's date of birth.			1	1
50. I find it very easy to play games with children that involve pretending.			1	1

GLOSSARY OF TERMS

Affective empathy: empathy towards people who we know are suffering (or who are victims of injustice).

AQ test: the abbreviation for the Autism Quotient test, which is for the initial screening of autism rather than diagnosis. This test was developed by Simon Baron-Cohen and other researchers from the Autism Research Centre in Cambridge, UK.

Aspergic (or Aspergerian): an adjective for someone who has AS.

Aspie: a colloquial term for a person who has AS.

Cognitive empathy (or theory of mind): the ability to perceive other people's thoughts and feelings.

Coming in: an idiom (arising from Aspergic 'wordplay') used by the author, meaning self-identification, and which is the beginning of the 'coming out' process.

Comorbidity: the coexistence of AS with another psychiatric condition (or disorder).

Dissociation: a psychiatric condition which causes the person to appear emotionally aloof or detached from people or events.

Dyspraxia: a developmental learning disability which causes difficulty with coordination and motor skills.

Medical model (of disability): a concept based on the belief that Aspergic people have a psychiatric disorder which needs to be cured. The disorder is deemed cured when the Aspergic person has learned to mimic neurotypical people. The medical model, which is aligned with cognitive behavioural therapy, causes most people on the spectrum to have poor mental health if they are not accepted by society.

Neurotypical: a term used by people who have AS to describe the ordinary ('normal') way of thinking; so a 'normal' person may be referred to as neurotypical.

Self-identification: the experience of realising our intellectual condition.

Social model (of disability): a concept based on the premise that people who have AS are potentially healthy, and therefore their environment should accept their differences to prevent the onset of mental ill health.

BIBLIOGRAPHY

American Psychiatric Association (APA) (2013) *Diagnostic and Statistical Manual of Mental Disorders (DSM-5)*. Arlington, VA: APA. Available at www. dsm5.org, accessed on 23 June 2013.

Asperger, H. (1944) *Autistic Psychopathy in Childhood* (in German). Republished in English in U. Frith (ed.) (1991) *Autism and Asperger Syndrome*. Cambridge: Cambridge University Press.

Attwood, T. (2006) *The Complete Guide to Asperger's Syndrome*. London: Jessica Kingsley Publishers.

Attwood, T. (2013) 'Ask Dr. Tony' *Autism Hangout Feature Programs*. Autism Hangout, 13 November 2013. Available online at www.autismhangout.com/news-reports/feature-programs.asp?id2=225.

Attwood, T. and Gray, C. (1999) 'The Discovery of Aspie Criteria.' *The Morning News, 11*, 3, 1–7.

Auyeung, B., Wheelwright, S., Allison, C., Atkinson, M., Samarawickrema, N. and Baron-Cohen, S. (2009) 'The Children's Empathy Quotient and Systemizing Quotient: Sex differences in typical development and in autism spectrum conditions.' *Journal of Autism and Developmental Disorders 39*, 1509–1521.

Baron-Cohen, S. (2008) *The Facts: Autism and Asperger's Syndrome*. Oxford: Oxford University Press.

Baron-Cohen, S. (2012) *Zero Degrees of Empathy: A New Theory of Human Cruelty and Kindness*. London: Penguin Books.

Baron-Cohen, S., Richler, J., Bisarya, D., Gurunathan, N. and Wheelwright, S. (2003) 'The Systemising Quotient (SQ): An investigation of adults with Asperger Syndrome or High Functioning Autism and normal sex differences.' *Philosophical Transactions of the Royal Society,* Series B (special issue), 358, 1430, 361–374.

Baron-Cohen, S., Robinson, D., Woodbury-Smith, M. and Wheelwright, S. (2007) *Very Late Diagnosis of Asperger Syndrome: The Cambridge Lifespan Asperger Syndrome Service (CLASS)*. Available at www.iancommunity.org/cs/articles/very_late_diagnosis_of_asperger_syndrome, accessed on 27 March 2013.

Beardon, L. (2007) *The Myths of Autism*. London: Asperger United.

Beardon, L. (2011) *Aspies on Mental Health*. London: Jessica Kingsley Publishers.

Bentley, K. (2007) *Alone Together: Making an Asperger Marriage Work*. London: Jessica Kingsley Publishers.

Birch, J. (2003) *Congratulations! It's Asperger Syndrome*. London: Jessica Kingsley Publishers.

Coojimanns, P. (2009) *Asperger's 1944 Article Summarized.* Available at www. paulcooijmans.com/asperger/asperger_summarized.html, accessed on 20 November 2012.

Debbaudt, D. (2002) *Autism, Advocates, and Law Enforcement Professionals: Recognizing and Reducing Risk Situations for People with Autism Spectrum Disorders.* London, UK: Jessica Kingsley Publishers.

Fitzgerald, M. (2006) *Andy Warhol and Konrad Lorenz: Two Persons with Asperger's Syndrome.* Available at http://professormichaelfitzgerald.eu/andy-warhol-and-konrad-lorenz-two-persons-with-aspergers-syndrome, accessed on 14 May 2014.

Frith, U. (1991) *Autism and Asperger Syndrome.* Cambridge: Cambridge University Press.

Gibbons, A. (1999) 'Mentoring definitions.' The Coaching and Mentoring Network. Available at www.coachingnetwork.org.uk/information-portal/Articles/ViewArticle. asp?artId=54, accessed on 24 May 2014.

Goldberg, M. and Berkman, J. (2013) *Sleep Problems in Children with Asperger Syndrome.* Asperger's Association of New England. Available at aane.org/ asperger_resources/articles/children_parenting/sleep_problems_asperger.html, accessed on 17 March 2013.

Goodyear, B. (2008) *Coaching People with Asperger's Syndrome.* London: KarnacBooks.

Grandin, T. (1990) *Emergence: Labeled Autistic.* New York: Grand Central Publishing (formerly Warner Books).

Jensen, K. (2012) 'Intelligence is overrated: What you really need to succeed.' *Forbes,* 4 December. Available at www.forbes.com/sites/keldjensen/2012/04/12/ intelligence-is-overrated-what-you-really-need-to-succeed, accessed on 24 March 2012.

Kanner, L. (1943) *Autistic Disturbances of Affective Contact.* Reprinted in A. M. Donnellan (ed.) (1985) *Classic Readings in Autism.* New York, NY: Teacher's College Press.

Kübler-Ross, E. (2005) *On Grief and Grieving: Finding the Meaning of Grief Through the Five Stages of Loss.* New York, NY: Simon & Schuster Ltd.

Lever, M. (2011) 'In the face of ignorance.' *Accountancy,* November, pp.98–99. London: CCH Editions.

Morris, R. and Wade, P. (2008) *Asperger's for Professionals.* Warwickshire: Wasp with Asperger Ltd.

Murray, D. (2006) *Coming Out Asperger: Diagnosis, Disclosure and Self-Confidence.* London: Jessica Kingsley Publishers.

Palmer, S. (2006) *Toxic Childhood: How the Modern World is Damaging Our Children and What We Can Do About It.* London: Orion Books Ltd.

Pitney Bowes International (1983) *Pitney Bowes Direct Sales training course.*

Plank, A. (2009) *Autism Reality* [Video]. Available at https://www.youtube.com/ watch?v=jLOCYubVc7g, accessed on 2 July 2014.

Rossiter, A. (2006) *Developing Spiritual Intelligence: The Power of You.* Winchester: O Books.

Sharamon, S. and Baginski, B. (1991) *The Chakra Handbook*. Twin Lakes, WI: Lotus Press.

Shay, K. (2010) 'What I Learned While Being Homeless.' Available at http://kylyssa. squidoo.com/homeless-experiences, accessed on 14 July 2014.

Silverman, L. K. (1993) *What is Giftedness?* Available at www.gifteddevelopment. com/What_is_Gifted/whatis.htm, accessed on 14 May 2014.

Wellyn, S. (2012) *Autistic Spectrum Disorder, MRI Brain Scan Diagnoses in Aspergers Autism.* Available at www.shazwellyn.hubpages.com/hub/Autistic-Spectrum-Disorder-Aspergers-Syndrome-Brain-Scan-Diagnoses-Autism, accessed on 22 December 2012.

Willingham, E. (2013) 'Autism prevalence is now at 1 in 50 children.' *Forbes*, 20 March. Available at forbes.com/sites/emilywillingham/2013/03/20/autism-prevalence-is-now-at-1-in-50-children, accessed 21 August 2013.

World Health Organization (2012) *International Classification of Diseases and Related Health Problems* (10th edn; *ICD-10*). Geneva: World Health Organization.

Wylie, P. and Heath, S. (2013) *VLDAS 2013 UK Survey*. Available at www. shropshireautonomy.co.uk/publications/survey-reports, accessed on 15 September 2013.

FURTHER READING

Aston, M. (2001) *The Other Half of Asperger Syndrome*. London: Jessica Kingsley Publishers.

Aston, M. (2003) *Asperger's in Love: Couple Relationships and Family Affairs*. London: Jessica Kingsley Publishers.

Aston, M. (2008) *The Asperger Couples Workbook: Making Difference Work*. London: Jessica Kingsley Publishers.

Aston, M. (2012) *What Men with Asperger's Want to Know About Women, Dating and Relationships*. London: Jessica Kingsley Publishers.

Brignell, V. (2010) 'The eugenics movement Britain wants to forget.' *The New Statesman,* 9 December. Available at www.newstatesman.com/society/2010/12/british-eugenics-disabled, accessed on 14 May 2014.

Guillebeau, C. (2010) *The Art of Non-Conformity*. London: Turnaround UK.

Hendrickx, S. (2008) *Love, Sex and Long-Term Relationships: What People with Asperger Syndrome Really Really Want*. London: Jessica Kingsley Publishers.

Hendrickx, S. (2008) *Asperger Syndrome and Employment: What People with Asperger Syndrome Really Really Want*. London: Jessica Kingsley Publishers.

Hendrickx, S. (2009) *The Adult and Adolescent Neuro-diversity Handbook*. London: Jessica Kingsley Publishers.

Hendrickx, S. and Needham, K. (2007) *Asperger Syndrome: A Love Story*. London: Jessica Kingsley Publishers.

Hendrickx, S. and Tinsley, M. (2008) *Asperger Syndrome and Alcohol: Drinking to Cope*. London: Jessica Kingsley Publishers.

Purkiss, J. and Royston-Lee, D. (2010) *Brand You: Turn Your Unique Talents into a Winning Formula*. London: Financial Times Guides.

Robinson, K. (2009) *The Element: How Finding Your Passion Changes Everything*. London: Penguin Books.

Wylie, P. (2014) *The Nine Degrees of Autism*. Available at www.latediagnosis-aspergers.pw, accessed on 14 May 2014.

INDEX

Lightning Source UK Ltd.
Milton Keynes UK
UKOW06f0942070415

249231UK00001B/17/P